Managing Nursing

Managing Nursing

A practical introduction to management for nurses

RAY ROWDEN SRN, RMN, Onc NC, MBIM
Director of Nursing Services
The Royal Marsden Hospital, Sutton, Surrey
Associate Editor, *The Nursing Times*

and the following contributors

PETER BREARLEY BA, RMN, RNMS, DN(London)
Regional Nurse, Planning
Oxford Regional Health Authority

JANICE CACKETT MSc, BA, SRN, DN, RNT
Director of Nurse Education
The Nightingale School of Nursing
St Thomas' Hospital, London

CHRISTINE HANCOCK SRN, BSc
Chief Nursing Officer, Bloomsbury Health Authority

DAVID MOSS MA, DMS, LHA, ACMA, IPFA
Finance Officer, East Dorset Health Authority

REGINALD PYNE SRN, RFN, FBIM
Principal Professional Officer
United Kingdom Central Council for Nursing
Midwifery and Health Visiting

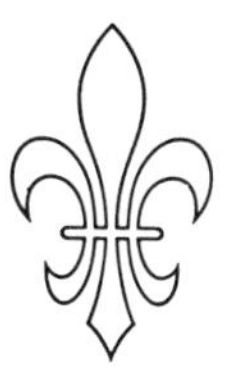

Baillière Tindall **London Philadelphia Toronto Mexico City Rio de Janeiro Sydney Tokyo Hong Kong**

Baillière Tindall 1 St Anne's Road
Eastbourne, East Sussex, BN21 3UN, England

W.B. Saunders West Washington Square
Philadelphia, PA 19105, USA

1 Goldthorne Avenue
Toronto, Ontario M8Z 5T9, Canada

Apartado 26370—Cedro 512
Mexico 4, DF, Mexico

Rua Evaristo da Veiga, 55–20° andar
Rio de Janeiro–RJ, Brazil

ABP Australia Ltd, 44 Waterloo Road
North Ryde, NSW 2064, Australia

Ichibancho Central Building, 22–1 Ichibancho
Chiyoda-ku, Tokyo 102, Japan

10/FL, Inter-Continental Plaza, 94 Granville Road
Tsim Sha Tsui East, Kowloon, Hong Kong

First published 1984

Typeset by Scribe Design, Gillingham, Kent
Printed in Great Britain by Biddles Ltd of Guildford

British Library Cataloguing in Publication Data

Rowden, Ray
Managing nursing.
1. Nursing service administration
I. Title
610.73'068 RT89

ISBN 0-7020-1047-2

Contents

About the Authors

This book has been prepared by authors who have a wide range of expertise in their fields

RAY ROWDEN has been actively involved in NHS industrial relations since 1971. As a practitioner, he was one of the first Rcn Stewards and wrote and lectured widely on the subject of nurses and industrial relations. He was elected to Rcn Council in 1977 and joined the staff of the Rcn in 1978, where he became Senior Officer to the Rcn Welsh Board, dealing mainly with advocacy and industrial relations. He was a member of the staff side of the Nurses and Midwives Whitley Council for two years, and a member of the Rcn Committee on Labour Relations for four years. He has also had experience as a member of a Community Health Council. Currently he is Director of Nursing Services at the Royal Marsden Hospital in Sutton and Associate Editor of *The Nursing Times*. He represents managers in the London Post-Graduate Teaching Hospitals on the National Executive Committee of the Rcn Association of Nursing Management.

PETER BREARLEY also worked as a full time staff member for the Rcn Welsh Board and has been a member of the Nurses and Midwives Whitley Council. He has had wide experience in training Rcn Stewards and was instrumental in designing training packages for Rcn Stewards and Safety Representatives in Wales. On leaving the Rcn he became Area Nurse Personnel for the Northamptonshire Area Health Authority. In 1983 he became Regional Nurse Planning for the Oxfordshire RHA.

JANICE CACKETT trained at The London Hospital, where she worked as a ward sister, tutor and senior tutor, prior to moving to her present post in 1977. She has a keen interest in the learning environment provided in the clinical situation and a commitment to staff development programmes. She has had wide experience in nurse education and has been a member of the General Nursing Council for England and Wales and of the Joint Board of

Clinical Nursing Studies. She was recently elected a member of the newly formed English National Board for Nursing, Midwifery and Health Visiting.

CHRISTINE HANCOCK has held a variety of senior appointments, including District Nursing Officer within the Camden and Islington Area Health Authority, prior to her present post as Chief Nursing Officer to the newly created Bloomsbury Health Authority. The creation of this new Inner London Health Authority posed some unique management problems, since it merged two of London's most famous teaching hospitals for management purposes, The Middlesex Hospital and University College Hospital. She has an active interest in the care of the elderly and is a member of the National Executive Committee of the Rcn Society of Geriatric Nursing. Miss Hancock was instrumental in pioneering the development of the role of Clinical Nursing Officer at Whipps Cross Hospital in the post-Salmon period. She is also a member of the Standing Nursing and Midwifery Advisory Committee.

DAVID MOSS has held a variety of posts in financial management in the NHS and has written widely on the subject. He is known throughout the U.K. for his creative and innovative work and is active within the Association of Health Service Treasurers. He has a keen interest in nursing and has written papers in conjunction with the Chief Nursing Officer in his Authority for a nursing readership. He is currently Finance Officer for the East Dorset Health Authority.

REGINALD PYNE has been closely involved with professional discipline over many years. Before his present appointment he was Deputy Registrar and Acting Registrar for the General Nursing Council for England and Wales, where he had responsibility for the functioning of the disciplinary committee. There can be no other nurse in the United Kingdom with his degree of experience in this field. He has been closely involved in the establishment of the new statutory framework arising out of the Nurses, Midwives and Health Visitors Act. He speaks widely on the subject of professional discipline and has written a bestseller on the subject. He is known for his sometimes controversial views on how the profession perceives itself and what it actually provides for the public and is an outspoken defender of clinical nurses who face stress in their working environment.

Preface

The marriage between nursing and management has not always been a harmonious one. In a relatively short period of time, nurses have had to come to grips with the modern approach to the running of a complicated service. It is, therefore, hardly surprising that many nurses still find difficulty in familiarising themselves with the art and science of management.

The aim of this book is to overcome some of those difficulties. In their day-to-day work all nurses manage, albeit to a varying degree. The nurse of today, and of the future, will be increasingly called upon to exercise control and perhaps, more importantly, account for decisions taken.

Management skills need to be developed at an early stage in the nurse's career if we are to produce nurses able to control the nursing service effectively. It must be remembered that nurses constitute the largest single professional group within health care. In any health authority, the nursing budget is likely to be the largest. This places enormous responsibilities on nurse managers.

Effective management of a large and expensive service is of vital importance and the skills involved are applicable to all nurses with a management role, be they ward sister or regional nursing officer.

If one begins to consider the amount of money and manpower required to run one ward, it becomes clear that the first line manager is directly responsible for controlling a substantial amount of resources and it is the quality of management at the first line level that will determine most of what the consumer experiences and do most to effect and influence the morale and performance of nursing personnel.

With these thoughts in mind, this book is written primarily for those managers in the first line and middle line level. I would hope that staff nurses preparing themselves for a ward sister's role and third year students undergoing a management module within their basic training might find sections of this book helpful.

The book can be read as a whole or individual chapters can be used for reference to particular subjects. Nursing and management have much in common: both are a balanced mixture of art and science, both are concerned primarily with getting the best out of people and both have an identical process. Just like the nurse, the wise manager is continually identifying problems or potential problems, setting goals, implementing action and evaluating the consequences of that action. Management, like nursing, demands similar skills. Like the nurse, the successful manager must be a good listener, a keen observer of human behaviour, have the ability to empathise and understand situations intelligently and, at times, make very difficult decisions under stress.

Nurses have all the basic raw material; the recipe for success is to mix basic nursing skills with a theoretical underpinning in the art and science of management.

There is, however, little point in nurses understanding the niceties of employment protection law until they can see the relevance of that law to their own working environment. Nurses are known to be practical people. I have, therefore, attempted to produce a text that is readable, easily understood and, above all, practically relevant to nurses and nursing.

There are many management textbooks on library shelves, but, so often, their style can appear to be somewhat dry and little has been written with nurses and nursing situations in mind. I hope that this book can go some way towards rectifying a deficit long recognised by many nurses.

RAY ROWDEN

Acknowledgements

The preparation of this manuscript involved a lot of hard work for a number of people. I would like to express thanks to my guest writers, all busy and eminent people. They had to tolerate my cajoling and all delivered first-rate chapters on time; without them the book would never have been published. I must thank Rosemary Long, Nursing Editor for Baillière Tindall, for her superb encouragement, patience and skill in steering the book from loose ideas in my head to the copy now in your hand.

I also thank the many friends and colleagues who allowed me to share ideas with them and who gave me the benefit of their views. Thanks are also due to Bob Tiffany, Chief Nursing Officer at the Royal Marsden Hospital, who allowed me the flexibility to complete the manuscript. Thanks to Pam Shrubshall, my long-suffering secretary, who did all of the typing. Finally, I thank the many nurses whom I have met over the years in times of difficulty. They have taught me an enormous amount on what management is about and the legislation related to employment.

Chapter 1
The History and Development of Management in Nursing

RAY ROWDEN

Nursing as a formally organised profession is relatively young, even though caring for the sick is as old as time itself. The concept of the nurse as a trained person was developed in the last century and registration for nurses was achieved in 1919 only after a long and hard battle. The idea of nurses managing nursing in a truly professional sense is younger still, dating probably from the early 1960s following the publication of the Salmon Report.

If we are to fully understand the position of the nurse in a managerial position today, we must look back to our history for there are many influences from our past that help us to understand how and why nursing management became what it is today.

THE EARLY YEARS

Nursing in the latter half of the 1800s was in a state of great change and turmoil. Florence Nightingale with her views on the needs of the profession was pre-eminent in shaping the destiny of nursing; she did not, however, have things all her own way. Ethel Bedford-Fenwick, whose ideas were opposed to Florence Nightingale's, also had a great deal of influence in developments leading up to the passing of the first nurses' act.

The arguments between these two ladies were at times bitter and acrimonious. The gestation and birth of modern nursing was long and, at times, extremely painful. Nursing had suffered from a very poor image in the earlier centuries, the profession lacked any organisation or formal training and few people had access to health care.

Nursing as a profession began to develop, with a few pioneering dominant women at the helm, at a time when the place of women in society was very strictly controlled and dominated by men. To understand the development of the control of nursing, it is vital to bear in mind the sociological backdrop against which these events were taking place, for it is evident that men, and in particular medical men, were able to exercise rigid control over nursing from the very beginning, and that they were to reign supreme for a very very long time. To a degree, this remains so today.

There are still many myths surrounding the handful of women who dominated the early development of the profession. Florence Nightingale, for example, is popularised as an angelic figure gently treading the wards of her military hospital in Scutari with lamp in hand, stroking the fevered brow of her patients, bringing all the traditionally feminine skills to the patient in need. The truth of the matter is very different. Florence Nightingale was a tenacious woman with political and administrative skill; for as a mere woman in Victorian society, she was able to bend the ears of cabinet ministers, doctors and other men in positions of power. In order to get her way, it is clear that she utilised harsh reality and pragmatism in support of her case. For example, she explained to the Secretary of State for War that adequate nursing at Scutari would get more soldiers back at the front, carrying guns. Ethel Bedford-Fenwick used similar methods to get her own way.

That these women achieved what they did was indeed remarkable. However, the fact remains that while they were instrumental in laying the foundations for the training and registration of nurses, they did little to challenge the basic assumption that men and doctors in particular were the only people fit to govern hospitals, almost by divine right.

An examination of contemporary literature bears this out time and time again. It must also be remembered that the women who followed Florence Nightingale into the upper echelons of nursing were mainly from upper middle class backgrounds, very far removed from the ancestry of the vast majority of women who actually staffed the wards. Paradoxically, nursing was not only externally influenced by the sexist attitudes prevalent within society at that time, it was also greatly influenced by class division within its own ranks.

This background laid the foundations for the nursing profession to become rigid and restricted, with ultimate control of its destiny removed from its own hands. In 1867, Henry Bonham-Carter wrote a pamphlet entitled *Suggestions for improving the management of the nursing departments of large hospitals*. The pamphlet makes interesting reading and in one section Bonham-Carter offers the following views on the office of Matron, 'the supreme position in the nursing hierarchy of the day':

> Under the present system in most of our hospitals, the Matron is the *nominal* chief of the nursing department. Her principal duties are, however, considered to be those of *housekeeping*, she is almost invariably selected for her qualifications in this respect.

> It rarely, if ever, happens that she has had any previous knowledge of the duties of nursing. The arrangement of any large hospital must be such that either the housekeeping duties are altogether separated from those of the superintendent of nurses, or that the matron or superintendent shall have an assistant as housekeeper.

The view expressed by Henry Bonham-Carter was to remain unchallenged for many years and it is clear from this that the scope for management of the nursing service in the sense that we know it today was extremely limited.

Henry Bonham-Carter was secretary to the Nightingale Fund which was used to finance the original system of nurse training at St Thomas' Hospital and it is interesting that a man so close to the venerable Florence Nightingale should hold such views of nursing management. It is also interesting to note his use of the term 'nominal chief of the nursing department' in connection with the office of Matron. Control of nursing practice rested very much in the hands of the doctor who implemented his wishes via the sister who usually ruled her domain in an autocratic fashion.

Documents of the period provide us with some fascinating insights into the régimes at ward level and into the flavour and scope of the matron's role. The nurse of the latter part of the nineteenth century was expected to be slavishly devoted to the gruelling work ethic. In the 1840s, nurses at St Thomas' Hospital received the grand sum of 19*s*.7*d*. per week plus a beer allowance. At St George's Hospital, nurses were paid £16.0*s*.0*d*. per annum, plus one shilling a day board allowance plus beer and bread. Sisters fared a little better in salary terms but were allowed the same beer and bread rations as ward nurses.

By the time the Nightingale School had been established at St Thomas' in the 1860s, salaries and conditions had improved very little, but women from a better social background who were recruited to the large London teaching hospitals were able to call on family support or were of independent financial means.

As the Nightingale model of training expanded, nursing became saturated with senior people from this type of background. Florence Nightingale ensured that her trainees were groomed for high office and many of the matrons of the large provincial hospitals and metropolitan hospitals were products of the School at St Thomas' Hospital. These women, in effect, could afford not to worry too much about salaries and conditions of service and many accepted the work ethic demanded of them. By 1887 women from the Nightingale School held positions of matron or superintendent of nursing at Westminster, Paddington, Marylebone, Highgate, Edinburgh, Huntingdon, Leeds, Lincoln, Liverpool, Southampton and Salisbury.

It is easy to see how Florence Nightingale spread her influence as widely as possible. It is also easy to see that she was exceedingly skilled in the art of delegation, for even when she took to her bed, she maintained a strong grip on the development of British nursing through her influence on others.

Autocratic management within nursing was accepted as the norm. The matrons in most hospitals did not have supreme power over the direction of their profession in that they were very much subservient within a well-defined hierarchy. The matron was perceived as being one rung below the hospital secretary, who in turn was one rung below the senior doctor. These women did, however, exercise great power over the lives and experiences of their staff and discipline was, in most hospitals, rigid. The correct wearing of uniform and the grooming of a nurse's hair are but two examples of the rigid control that was exercised, and vestiges of this habit are still to be found today.

The majority of probationers, ward nurses and sisters also lived in their hospitals, often close to ward areas, and their personal and private lives were also very much under the eye of the matron and her assistants.

Management in this environment was, to say the least, an uncomplicated affair when measured against the role of the manager today. The power to make decisions about financial matters, the planning of services and often the selection and recruitment of nursing staff were all vested outside the matron's direct control.

To a large degree, the greater part of the matron's role was concerned with controlling the day-to-day lives of the staff and ensuring that the standard of housekeeping within the hospital was adequate. There is no doubt that many illustrious women had wider vision and aspired to greater things and it is to these women that nursing owes a debt of gratitude for the degree of professional independence that is enjoyed today.

Women like Dame Sarah Swift, matron of Guy's Hospital at the turn of the century, Rachel Cox-Davies, matron of the Royal Free Hospital, and Alicia Lloyd-Still, matron of St Thomas' Hospital, were all powerful personalities who passionately believed in the development of nursing as a profession in its own right. All had either links or sympathies with the women's movement for emancipation. It is clear, however, that in the battle to achieve greater professional status for nursing, they all had to work through men who were either eminent doctors or administrators.

The die for a style of nursing management was, therefore, cast very early on in the professional development of nursing. Trade unionism among nurses was virtually unheard of until relatively recently and the hierarchy both in a sexist and in a professional sense has remained largely accepted and unchallenged throughout this century.

THE FORMATIVE YEARS

In the UK, the provision of formalised training for nurses in managerial positions developed slowly. The Royal College of Nursing set up its first one-year course for nurse administrators in 1944, but this course was very much viewed as being for potential matrons and scope for formalised training in management and administration outside London remained limited. Formalised preparation for responsibilities in middle management grades remained virtually non-existent until the mid-1960s. In the USA, college-based management courses for nurses began much earlier and literature related to the subject developed more rapidly.

The year 1966 proved to be a milestone in the management of nursing in the UK. A committee appointed by the then Minister of Health under the chairmanship of Brian Salmon published its report on the senior management structure of the nursing service.

Prior to 1966, the management of nursing had been under the auspices of the accepted hierarchical chain, that is, doctor, group secretary, matron/chief male nurse. The matron often did not have access to the hospital management committee and had to go to the supreme managing authority through the group secretary. In many settings, the matron/chief male nurse had to report formally to the group secretary for the management of the nursing service.

In reality, this meant the crucial policy decisions related to nursing could be, and often were, overruled by the group secretary and medical superintendent within the hospital. In the community services, health was under the direction of local authorities who each appointed their own chief medical officer and chief executive officer. In many areas, the director of community nursing was managerially subservient to both the chief medical officer and the county chief executive officer. In other words, the system of management in hospital was replicated almost exactly in the community services.

The Salmon Report recognised that the time had come to radically alter the pattern of management. The report recommended the creation of new grades in first, middle and top line management and created the post of chief nursing officer to all hospital management committees. The emphasis on the acquisition of appropriate management skills was emphasised throughout the new posts and Salmon laid the foundations which were to free nursing from managerial dominance by other professions.

Since 1966, many myths have evolved around the original proposals of the Salmon Report and one was that the new structure creamed off the best ward sisters into an army of 'pen-pushing', non-productive nurse administrative grades. The myths were perpetuated by doctors and administrators who clearly had some interest in maintaining the status quo. These myths were challenged in the report of the Royal Commission on the National Health Service in 1979 which showed that the numbers of nurses in management grades had actually decreased in the period between the advent of the Salmon proposals and the Commission's report.

There have without doubt been many teething problems in developing nurses as managers in a professional sense. Salmon's multi-tiered hierarchical structure, with much blurring of roles, was not an easy system to introduce. However, nurses have Salmon to thank for realising the value of professional management in a service as large, expensive and complex as nursing.

In the community services, a committee similar to Salmon's was established at about the same time under the chairmanship of Mayston. The authors of the Mayston report also accepted the philosophy of nurses managing nursing and a new structure was introduced within the local authority nursing services. The National Health Service realised that the new managerial roles created by Salmon required a great deal of training and preparation that had hitherto not been available. To this end, plans were laid to expand the availability of management training and education for nurses in the first, middle and top line grades.

Unfortunately, in many areas the cart was put before the horse in that many hospital management committees introduced new management structures with little or no preparation for post holders or potential post holders. For this reason, many of the early chief nursing officers were thrust into a game that they could not fully understand.

THE DEVELOPMENT OF NURSING MANAGEMENT

The demand for new skills

It is clear, then, that nursing managed by nurses got off to a shaky start. However, the seeds had been sown and training opportunities grew during the late 1960s and early 1970s. Many imaginative hospital management committees allowed the development of first line management courses on an in-service basis. Some also allowed their chief nursing officers to attend top line management courses, often multi-professional and based in universities and other institutes of higher education. This began an exposure of some of our top nurses to the world of professional management at a very senior level and was to have wide-ranging effects on the future patterns and styles of management at that level.

The availability of training remained patchy and it was to be many years before the statutory bodies controlling nurse education built into the training syllabuses of the registered nurse a formalised management module to be studied during the third year of training. In 1972, six years after the Salmon Report, the report of the Committee on Nursing, chaired by Asa Briggs, said of the Salmon structure:

> The Salmon Report which set out to raise nursing from 'the secondary position which it seemed to occupy' introduced a new structure in nursing and midwifery. The structure is headed by a chief nursing officer – a new post responsible direct to the governing body for all the nursing and midwifery services including education within a group of hospitals. In Chapter 6 of our report we discuss the particular aspects of this structure and make a number of recommendations concerning new posts in clinical nursing and midwifery and in nursing and midwifery education. We have preferred throughout our report to talk of duties and responsibilities rather than in terms of numbered Salmon grades and we have tried to extend recognition of clinical and educational duties and responsibilities as well as managerial duties and responsibilities. We are in full agreement with the Salmon committee, however, in pressing for increased participation by nurses and midwives in decision-making processes, and we welcome the genuine improvements which have been brought about in practice as the Salmon Report has been put into operation.

Briggs, therefore, fully accepted the philosophy that was inherent within the Salmon proposals. However, in the same section of the report, the committee goes on to say: '...we have noted that it seems likely that by 1972/73 all hospital groups will have appointed a chief nursing officer, or where appropriate a principal nursing officer, and that many groups will also have appointed all their senior grades.' From this it can be seen that change within nursing structures was slow and in actuality it did indeed take until 1973 for all hospital groups to appoint chief nursing officers.

This pattern was repeated in the community nursing services and Table 1, taken from the Briggs report, gives some indication of the slow progress in accepting and implementing the recommendations of the Mayston report.

Briggs recognised the importance of skilled management and critically examined the role of management in Chapter 6 of the report of the Committee on Nursing. Prior to the reorganisation of the National Health Service in 1974, Briggs had this to say about extending the type of management positions in nursing:

> Within the organisation of line management, nurses and midwives from every field should be given opportunities to reach the top. At the top, chief nurses within line management will cover a wider span of responsibility than ever before and may need, at area level at least, to call on the help in a staff capacity of specialist advisers in fields

Table 1 Implementation of the Mayston report.

	Position as at 31.12.1970	Position as at 27.3.1972	Position as at 20.7.1972
Total number of local health authorities (England)	158	158	158
Number of Directors of Nursing Services in post	107	124	132
Number of authorities who have made proposals	57	138	147
Formal or informal agreement given	4	105	125
Schemes fully implemented	—	27	51
Schemes partially implemented	—	34	42

which are unfamiliar to them. Outside line management, therefore, we see scope for a fuller development of staff posts at senior levels requiring special expertise of different kinds. All nurses and midwives should, so far as possible, have the opportunity of specialising in a particular subject if they desire and in each case their work could span hospital and community care.

Many of the Briggs recommendations were to influence the development of the profession in a wide-ranging sphere of activities, not least in the field of management.

The idea of specialist nurse managers supporting top line managers was to be one part of the proposals of the 1974 reorganisation of the National Health Service. It was not, of course, purely the Briggs proposals that brought about this development. At the time of the 1974 reorganisation, the government of the day was considering, or had already implemented, new employment legislation which was making the relationship between the employer and the employee much more complex in law and the health service was, of course, not exempt from this trend.

Employment legislation greatly influenced industrial society and covered matters such as health and safety at work, trade union rights, maternity benefit, dissemination of information to workers, contract law, race relations, etc. These developments radically influenced the climate of industrial relations within the health service generally and in the nursing service specifically. As the body of law related to industrial relations grew, it became increasingly obvious that the top line manager could not devote the necessary time and attention to fully understanding its implications for the management of a service as large and complex as nursing. This, probably more than anything else, forced the nursing service to consider the need for specialist support posts at senior level in management.

Trade unionism

The other major factor to influence the development and style of management within the nursing service has been the influence of trade unions within the service.

It is not surprising that the first influences of trade unionism within health care were to be found in the psychiatric service. In 1912, the National Asylum Workers Union was battling against a working week for men and women which was often in excess of 70 hours exclusive of meal times, and in some cases, 80 or 90 hours a week. Asylum attendants were also expected to live in the wards, almost 'on top of their job', so that they were, in effect, on call at all times. General salary levels were equally appalling. The public perception of asylum workers was extremely poor and contemporary records bear this out. In the face of these conditions and the general image of the asylum worker, it is hardly surprising that workers looked to the organisation of the labour force with a view to beginning a struggle to improve their lot. Trade unionism within asylums had begun in the late 1800s and early 1900s, but contemporary records show that there was a great argument involving those within society who wanted to emphasise the professionalism of the work of the nurse and to place the importance of salaries and conditions of service in a secondary place.

There were more men than women in the workforce of the asylums and this was undoubtedly influential in the development of the trade union movement within the nursing service. This is probably due to the fact that because of the large degree of sex-stereotyping, men had to make an economically viable career within the nursing service and were, therefore, under more urgent pressure to improve their financial lot and their working conditions generally.

Prior to generalised employment legislation in the mid-1970s, there was a great reluctance on the part of many nurses to identify with the aspirations of the trade union movement generally. The Royal College of Nursing itself did not become certified as an independent trade union until well into the 1970s and even then, only after great debate within its membership. The College remains outside the TUC and committed to a policy of 'no strike' and it is clear that much conflict remains in the minds of nurses in relation to the role of a trade union.

Contemporary records related to pay bargaining during the 1930s, 1940s and 1950s show quite clearly that this conflict had a real influence on the climate of pay bargaining during these decades. The College continually advanced reasons related to professionalism which were to hold nursing to a more moderate position in the pay bargaining stakes.

However, it must be recognised that nursing membership within the generic trade unions to some degree shared these conflicts and even up to the present day, most nurses appear to be in agreement with a 'no strike' posture in the industrial relations scene.

The legislation of the 1970s, however, not only forced nurse managers to reappraise their role and function, but also made the nursing organisations examine themselves.

In 1971, when the Conservative government of the day introduced the first industrial relations act, the Royal College of Nursing, followed shortly after by some of the other professional organisations, began to recognise the need for the provision of a shop-floor service to members related to industrial-relations-style activities. To this end, an Rcn stewards scheme was commenced where local members were trained fully in recruitment, problem handling, grievance handling and general industrial representation. From this period the scheme took off dramatically and it is evident that the members, while not necessarily identifying with traditional industrial concepts, were very appreciative of the development of a stewards scheme at local level.

Nurses' pay has always been a highly centralised bargaining issue. However, as I explain in later chapters in this book, many other issues concern nurses, for example, local conditions of work, rules and regulations related to disciplinary matters, and health and safety at work. It is probably in these areas that we have seen the greatest influences from the trade unions on management at the local level. Tensions and conflicts no doubt remain, but the number of nurses joining trade unions and organisations and becoming active has increased and continues to do so. As nurses began gradually to identify more with their needs as workers in the general hospital setting, more problems were posed for nurse managers.

Higher education

One other great influence on the development of nursing management has been the gradual acceptance of degree-level education for nurses. In the last decade we have seen an enormous rate of growth in the number of universities and institutes of higher education offering degree-level education to nursing staff. At the same time, there has been a growth in the number of degree-level courses in management sciences. The number of nurses who are able to undertake degrees related to business, financial management and public sector administration continues to grow. This pattern of preparation continues to expose nurses at the top to a broader range of influences and will undoubtedly do much to influence the style and scope of nursing management in the future. There is without doubt a long way to go and there is still a great deal to learn about the concept of management in teams. But when one examines the nursing profession's ancestry and lineage, it is really quite remarkable how far the profession has travelled in a relatively short span of time when compared to other professional groups.

Team management

The concept of team management at senior level is relatively new, having been formally introduced during the 1974 reorganisation of the service. In 1983 the concept was introduced at unit level in both community and hospital services. This development is entirely logical and it is right and proper that nurses as managers should be seen to operate in teams of equals on the same terms in relation to their influence on general health care provision within the local health authority. This philosophy has been challenged by the report of Roy Griffiths to the Conservative Secretary of State for Health, published in November 1983. This report suggests that general managers be appointed throughout the service. It is possible that a number of nurses would become general managers.

Team management, if carried out, will place increasing demands on the manager at unit level and the staff who work within the unit in managerial grades. Nurses as specialist managers will also need to be flexible in their response to a changing managerial climate. Manpower planning, capital planning, personnel services and new technology pose managers with the need for increased development and training opportunities. There is also going to have to be a critical examination of the kind of preparation that is available for the senior nurses, directors of nursing services and chief nursing officers of the future, since there now seems to be a greater emphasis within the profession on developing clinical career structures as opposed to limiting career opportunities to managerial and teaching grades.

If this trend continues, it is clear that fewer nurses will be choosing management or education as a career option. Well-prepared professional managers who are also nurses are going to be essential for the success of any enterprise engaged in health care. It is, therefore, vital that the nursing profession keeps under constant review the preparation that it offers to its potential managers of the future.

Suggested further reading

Abel-Smith, B. (1960) *The History of the Nursing Profession*. London: Heinemann.

Bellaby, P. & Oribabor, P. (1977) The growth of trade union consciousness among general hospital nurses. *Sociological Review*, Vol. 25, pp. 801–822.

Bendall, E. & Raybould, E. (1970) *A History of the General Nursing Council for England & Wales 1919–1969*. London: H.K. Lewis.

Bowman, G. (1967) *The Lamp and the Book—A History of the RCN*. London: Royal College of Nursing.

Cowell, B. & Wainwright, D. (1981) *Behind the Blue Door: A History of the RCM 1881–1981*. London: Baillière Tindall.

Davies, C. (ed.) (1981) *Re-Writing Nursing History*. London: Croom Helm. (See particularly Chapter 2, Nurse recruitment to four provincial hospitals 1881 –1921, by Christopher Maggs; Chapter 3, From Sarah Gamp to Florence Nightingale. A critical study of hospital nursing systems from 1840–1897, by Katherine Williams; Asylum nursing before 1914. A chapter in the history of nursing labour, by Mick Carpenter; Chapter 7, The history of the present contradiction and struggle in nursing', by Paul Bellaby & Patrick Oribabor.)

Hector, W. (1973) *Mrs Bedford-Fenwick*. London: Royal College of Nursing.

Mayston Report (1966) London: HMSO.

Newby, M.S. (1976) *Florence Nightingale—A Woman of All Time, Myths and Stereotypes*. Society for the Social History of Medicine, Bulletin 18.

Report of an Inquiry into the management of the Health Service to the Secretary of State (1983) London: HMSO.

Report of the Committee on Nursing (Briggs) (1972) London: HMSO.

Report of the Committee on Senior Nursing Staff Structure (Salmon) (1966) London: HMSO.

Report of the Royal Commission on the National Health Service (1979) Chairman Sir Alex Merrison. London: HMSO. (See particularly Appendix H, Evidence from the Advisory, Conciliation and Arbitration Service, pp. 457–469.)

White, R. (1978) *Social Change and the Development of the Nursing Profession*. London: Henry Kimpton.

Chapter 2
What is Management?

RAY ROWDEN

Defining management in neat clichés is rather a waste of time. There is argument in the ranks of management as there is in the ranks of nursing about what management is or is not, and about whether or not it can be described as a profession, controlling its own destiny and standards and possessing a unique, definable body of knowledge. These arguments will continue, but the manager in today's Health Service needs to keep an open mind and to be aware of a host of different ideas, attitudes and theories about the subject.

One thing is absolutely certain: no-one can state exactly what constitutes 'good' or 'bad' management. No-one can yet define authoritatively what is a right or a wrong way of managing. Typical management, therefore, is an unreal concept. Management in all its forms is a question of individual style, running from the extreme autocrat at one end of the scale to the extreme democrat at the other end, with a host of variable styles in between.

The question of what is right or wrong is a matter of individual judgement. What one can say, however, is that all managers should understand quite clearly what they are doing and why they are doing it. To manage blindly, with little or no insight into one's actions, is, to say the least, a risky approach to take. Against the background of uncertainty within the field of management, there is an enormous amount of valuable social, economic and psychological research which has been undertaken and much of this work has relevance to managers in all enterprises, including nursing.

In this chapter, I would like to examine the more commonly known and accepted research related to management practice with a view to stimulating further reading and perhaps encouraging a willingness to develop greater personal insight on the part of the individual nurse manager into his/her own conduct.

The concept of nurses managing nursing in a truly professional sense is relatively young. The preparation for becoming a manager in the nursing service has been, and to a great extent still is, extremely poor. Many nurse managers in senior positions today have worked their way up through the ranks with little or no specialised training. This is rather like asking a neuro-surgeon to successfully manage a gang of labourers laying a new motorway from Land's End to John O'Groats – it is doomed to failure!

The training model in nursing is geared heavily towards the acquisition of clinical skills; this is, of course, as it should be. But once the nurse qualifies, much of the limited management training that is available is insular, often being uni-disciplinary and based within National Health Service institutions. For this reason, many nurses who hold management positions are never exposed to the broader information which is available to assist them in their work.

Professional management is also a relatively young concept. However, formalised social research into people at work and into management began as far back as 1911, when Gilbreth undertook some early studies into man at work.

One of the commonly held views in management circles during the industrial revolution and in the early part of this century was that money was the major motivating factor in the performance of people at work. On this basis, motivation is reported to consist of knowing how to dangle money as artfully as possible before the workforce. The carrot-and-stick theory of management is one of the oldest in existence and is based largely on assumptions about people that have now been challenged by behavioural scientists. Effective management was thought to be a rather simple and straightforward affair. Many managers held the basic view that man was inherently lazy, despised work and worked only in the hope of making a lot of money, or in the fear of losing the chance to make any at all. Management, therefore, simply consisted of paying enough money to arouse people's greed, but not enough to spoil them.

As society became more heavily industrialised and operations became implemented on a larger and larger scale, employing more people and plant, greater management skills were required. This led to a number of pioneers in the field of social research examining what motivated people at work and how best to maximise the factors which motivate people.

RESEARCH INTO MOTIVATION

One of the earliest pieces of research into motivation at work was undertaken in the USA in the 1920s and is known as 'the Hawthorne Experiment'. The research was carried out at the Hawthorne works of a large electronic company where telephone equipment was made. The management of the company wanted to understand more about the factors that affected the performance of their workers and they asked the National Research Council of the National Academy of Sciences to carry out some research.

The study was concerned with finding out what sort of physical conditions affected work. After preliminary studies between 1924 and 1927, the researchers selected a group of girls involved in the assembly of telephone relays. The work involved was routine and repetitive and in order to study the effects of physical conditions more easily, a sub-group of six girls was moved to a separate room away from the main group. The sub-group was then closely observed at work and accurate records of actual output were kept. Soon after the move, various changes were made in the length of hours worked, starting and finishing times and the number of rest periods given, and control was exercised over what the girls ate during their working day.

The study lasted from 1927 until 1929 and found that, despite the changes that were made in the physical environment, output amongst the girls steadily increased. The changes made were both favourable and unfavourable to the girls concerned, but still output increased. This phenomenon is known as 'the Hawthorne Effect' and was explained in the following way. It was thought that the girls in the sub-group were responding mainly to the fact that they were being identified for a study and, therefore, perceived that they were receiving special treatment. The girls separated from the main assembly room were given better working conditions than the main group. They became involved and interested in the study and were kept informed of the changes that were taking place at each stage of the project. They also developed a rapport with the research workers. Following this study, the researchers and the company expanded their ideas, and between 1928 and 1931, 21,000 employees were interviewed about their work and their reactions to it.

This study made available a massive amount of reliable data related to motivation and work. The researchers also went on to do more work with a controlled group of 14 men which revealed some fascinating information about group behaviour and its influences at work.

Other researchers have studied the data obtained during the Hawthorne studies and it is accepted by many that this early work was very important in the development of our understanding of the relationship between man and his work.

The studies supported the move from more traditional mechanistic management styles to a more progressive outlook based on the view that motivation is a far more complex subject than had previously been realised.

Another researcher with an interest in the psychology of motivation was

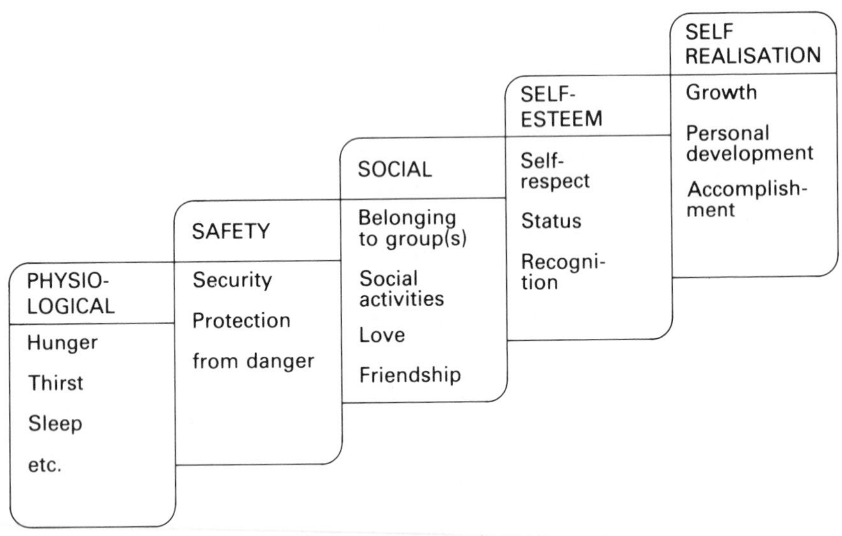

Figure 1. Man's basic needs.

Abraham Maslow, who in 1954 defined a hierarchy of people's needs. Based on extensive clinical studies, Maslow set a classification of at least five sets of goals which he called 'man's basic needs'. These are shown in Figure 1. Maslow felt that these needs tend to have to be satisfied in a given order and that once a lower order of need is satisfied, either totally or partially, the aims and drives of a person will shift to those appropriate to a higher order of needs and that some of the lower order of needs may become less significant in this process. The needs can be summarised as follows:

1. *Physiological needs* – the needs of food, drink, warmth and shelter, etc.; that is, needs at a basic physiological level of function.
2. *Safety and security needs* – the need for stability in life. Protection, freedom from anxiety or chaos, the need to understand an order or structure and freedoms and limitations in situations. These lead the individual to desire job security, routine, good conditions of service, etc.
3. *Social* – if the above needs are met, the individual then realises the need to belong and to be loved within the family or within the work setting, that is, to avoid feeling lonely or out on a limb.
4. *Esteem needs* – these needs stem from our basic desire not to feel helpless or inferior. They are related to wanting to have a reasonably high evaluation of ourselves, that is, to like oneself. Self-esteem and to like others.

Maslow classified these needs into two definable sets:

(a) The desire for competence and achievement in the face of life at work and in general, and for a feeling of personal independence and freedom.

(b) The desire for prestige and esteem from others, status or fame, that is, to be appreciated. The failure to meet these needs successfully leads to feelings of inferiority or weakness, leading to discouragement or neurotic trends in order to compensate.

5. *The need for self-actualisation* – simply, this is the need for an individual to realise his full potential, that is, the desire for self-fulfilment.

   Maslow suggested that self-actualising people tend to be propelled by a gross motivation rather than by a deficiency motivation.

Maslow's hierarchy is often interpreted very rigidly in a fixed predictable order. Others have suggested that this is unwise. Maslow himself recognised that there are some people for whom self-esteem, for example, is far more important than love. However, his work is vital in terms of how we understand and consider people at work. Maslow indicated the value and importance of satisfying higher needs within work settings. He showed us that while the physical and social environments in which a job is done are of importance, of equal importance is the content of the job itself, something which was, and still is, neglected by many managers.

Another well-known researcher in the field of motivation theories is Professor Frederick Herzberg of Cleveland, Ohio, who carried out studies in the 1950s. Herzberg asked a group of engineers and accountants to describe how they felt in detail at times when they were particularly happy and settled in their jobs. Conversely, he asked them how they felt when their job situation was far from satisfactory or was frustrating. He found that factors affecting levels of satisfaction and dissatisfaction were not simple opposites, but that they had their source in different areas of the work situation, and that the removal of a dissatisfying factor from work did not necessarily have the assumed effect of increasing satisfaction levels. Herzberg defined this as the 'motivation/hygiene theory'. The factors Herzberg identified were:

Major dissatisfiers – causing low morale and low performance
(in ranked order)
Company policy and administration
Supervision and technical matters
Salary
Interpersonal relations/supervision
Working conditions

Major motivators – causing high morale and high performance
(in ranked order)
Sense of achievement
Recognition
Work itself
Responsibility
Advancement
Salary

What is striking about Herzberg's findings is that salary is given a very low priority as either a motivator or a dissatisfier. This would suggest that managers in a low-pay area such as nursing should be able to pay attention to non-pay factors in order to achieve maximum performance from their staff.

Herzberg questions the basic assumption that removal of dissatisfiers in itself will lead to job satisfaction, which, in turn, should lead to increased performance. The 'motivation/hygiene theory' turns this assumption on its head and suggests that it is more likely that good performance will lead to job satisfaction and that good performance can only occur where the characteristics of jobs are changed to allow a sense of autonomy and fulfilment of potential by the individual.

However, Walker and Guest, studying assembly line workers in 1957, found that the opposite was true. In this study it was found that workers were more satisfied by factors associated with pay and job security and that sources of discontent lay in the job context factors, for example, the setting of the level of work by an assembly line.

It is, of course, possible that different levels of occupation are influenced by totally different motivating factors. An engineer or an accountant may not have seen money as an important factor because the majority were relatively well paid in contrast to an assembly line worker, who would naturally place greater emphasis on pay and related conditions.

RESEARCH INTO MANAGING PEOPLE

Another social researcher whose views are well accepted is Douglas MacGregor, who argued in his book *The Human Side of Enterprise* that management is a profession because it possesses a unique and established body of scientifically based knowledge on which management practices can and should be based. He argued that one of management's major functions is to organise human effort in an attempt to meet the managerial objectives of the

Figure 1.

enterprise concerned. This depends on the manager having the ability to predict and control human behaviour and interaction at work.

MacGregor examined different theories related to behaviour in the working environment and developed two models which he called 'Theory X' and 'Theory Y'.

Theory X assumes that:

1. The average person dislikes work and will seek to avoid it where possible.
2. Because of an inherent dislike of work, most people need to be controlled and threatened before they will perform effectively.
3. Most people actually prefer to be led, dislike responsibility, are lacking in ambition and like and need security above all else.

'Theory X' assumptions are responsible for an organisational philosophy which is based on the 'be tough' management style with punishments and tight controls. This approach is also responsible for the 'be soft' philosophy which aims for harmony in the work setting. MacGregor felt that both these approaches based on Theory X were wrong because they overlook the fact that man needs more than financial rewards at work. He needs a higher order of motivation with the opportunity of maximum self-fulfilment. 'Theory X' managers are unable to facilitate this process of fulfilment and their employees, therefore, behave in the expected fashion, almost producing a self-fulfilling prophecy based on the manager's own philosophy and style.

Theory Y assumes that:

1. Physical and psychological effort applied in a work setting is a completely natural process.
2. The application of control and punishment is not necessarily the only way to make people perform well; man is capable of self-direction if he is committed to the overall goals of the organisation in which he is employed.
3. If the job itself is satisfying, this will result in the development of commitment to the organisation.
4. With the right environment and conditions, most people can learn to accept and also to seek responsibility on a personal level.
5. Creativity and imagination can be used to solve problems at work, even by large numbers of employees.

6. In our modern, technologically biased society, the intellectual and academic capabilities of the average employee are rarely fully utilised.

These assumptions arise from social science research which has been carried out over many years and which demonstrates the potential which all men possess and which managers need to recognise in order to be fully effective.

MacGregor saw these theories not as two opposite ends of a continuum, but as two distinct approaches to management. He showed in his work how Theory Y is difficult to apply in large mass-production-style industries, but argues that it can initially be applied in the management of professional people within such a setting.

He also saw Theory Y as a basis for a participative problem-solving approach to management. In certain settings, MacGregor accepted that authoritarian management styles based on Theory X were needed, particularly where subordinate staff either disagreed with, or did not understand, the overall goals of the organisation. However, where it is possible to obtain understanding and commitment to objectives, it is desirable that management explain matters carefully and completely in order that employees understand the purpose of management's actions.

MacGregor also argued that this approach would then encourage self-direction and lead to better work performance. He felt that management, once persuaded that it is underestimating the potential of its workforce, can then understand Theory Y assumptions and take the time and trouble in developing the application of the theory.

He recognised the weakness of his arguments, but made a plea that managers should apply in practical terms the basic assumption that employees will contribute more and perform more efficiently if they are treated as responsible and valued people.

RESEARCH INTO THE MANAGER'S ROLE

In an attempt to define in clear terms what constitutes the role of the manager, two researchers – Dr R. Blake and Dr J. Mouton – developed the managerial grid which reached this country in 1965 and has been accepted by many management teams as part of their training programmes. The grid is a method of examining existing research in the field of behavioural science and provides a framework which the individual manager can use to examine himself and his organisation (Figure 2). The grid is a simple chart with the horizontal axis presenting concern for production or performance on a

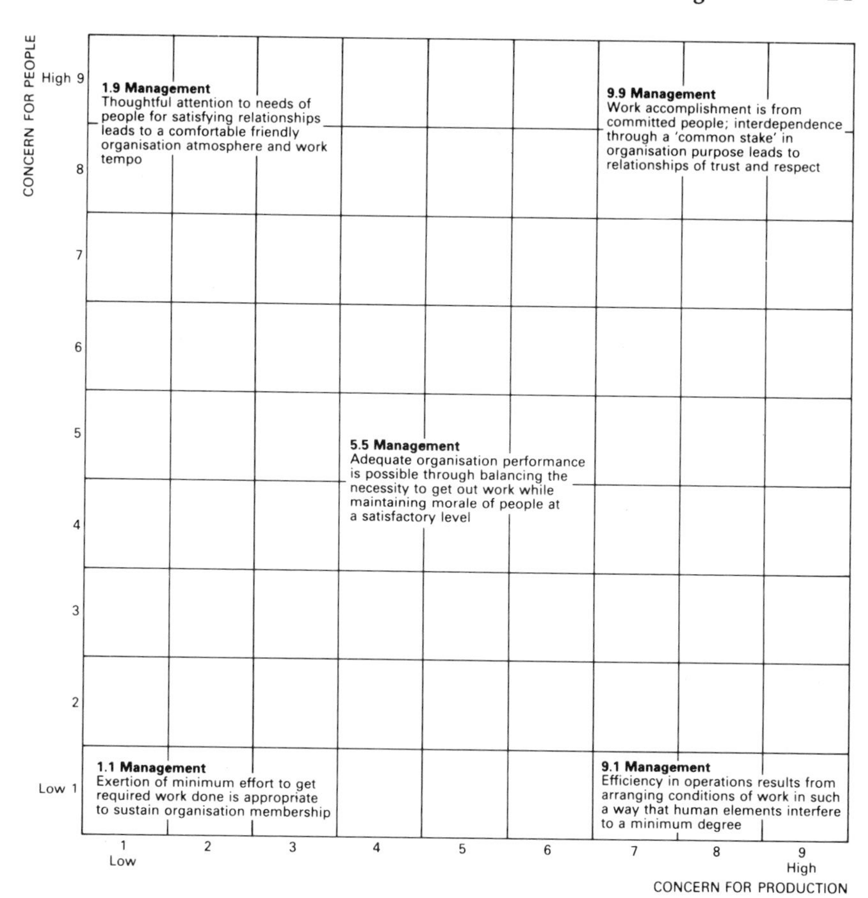

Figure 2. The managerial grid.

nine-point scale of values. The vertical axis represents the amount of concern for personnel that the manager has on the same nine-point scale. It can be used to demonstrate in clear terms the interests between what the grid theory defines as the three universals in any organisation, that is, people, production of goods or provision of services and hierarchy.

Theoretically, there are 81 positions which can describe a manager's behaviour or system. One can plot on the grid the point where a manager's concern for people matches up to his concern for production of the service and one should be able to identify his managerial style.

Blake and Mouton felt that management style comprised two elements: the practical side, involving itself with provision of service or production of goods, and the human, personnel-related element. The practical element involves itself with methods of decision-making, the control of employees being related to the efficient provision of a service. The personnel factors involve the manager in having an interest in matters such as conflict, emotion, humour, expression of ideas, all of which are related to interpersonal relationships within the work setting.

DELEGATION IN MANAGEMENT

The successful manager is involved in achieving his own objectives through the work of others. For this to happen effectively, the manager must be able to delegate. Delegation involves giving responsibility to others who should be responsible to the manager for results achieved. To delegate efficiently, the manager must apply some basic rules:

He must explain and define in clear terms the objective or task and ensure that it is understood by the officer or officers to whom the task is delegated.
He must also delegate the necessary authority to staff in order that they can meet the objectives or perform the tasks delegated.
He must attempt to match the task to the right person in the management team.
He must ensure effective communication and should always aim to encourage discussion of ideas and problems.
He should always establish proper control over delegated areas of work. This requires a sensitive approach, for there is a real danger that a manager can oversupervise. The wise manager should not be giving the impression that he is 'breathing down people's necks', for if he has to adopt this approach, it is a reflection on his own poor skills and lack of judgement.

A balance is needed, for there is an equal danger in the delegation of tasks or objectives with inadequate controls. The manager must choose areas of work that can be delegated judiciously and with care.
The manager should decide what are the major issues involving policy which cannot be delegated and equally should identify the trivial or routine matters that can and properly should be given to others.
He should always attempt to reward good performance by positive praise or encouragement.

Efficient delegation has many advantages. It can extend the manager's capacity and allow him to concentrate his efforts on the matters that count, leaving more time for overall planning and direction within his area of responsibility. Delegation can also engender a greater sense of fulfilment in subordinate personnel who are able to feel effectively in control of an area of activity. Delegation also allows for decisions to be taken nearer to the shop floor.

Wise delegation can also be used as an effective means of developing the management skills and aptitudes of junior staff in a useful and constructive way.

CONCLUSIONS

Management is a mixture of art and science. While it is true that there is a wealth of research on which to base management practices, there are many areas that are not clearly defined. In simple terms, there is little that is absolutely black or absolutely white, only varying shades of grey.

To a great extent, management can be based on scientific principles and people at work can be predictable. However, if all management styles were clearly and absolutely defined, there would be little room for the use of flair, imagination and instinctive judgement in the manager's life. The wise manager, therefore, needs to combine a sound knowledge of management sciences with an application of that knowledge in an open-minded way in his day-to-day work.

Additionally, he needs to recognise the importance of himself as a human and the effects he has on his work. All managers have their strengths and weaknesses, their likes and dislikes, their own unique prejudices, all of which influence their own performance and judgements. The manager who possesses a vast encyclopaedic knowledge of scientific research but who fails to acquire any insight into his own personality is, in my view, doomed to failure. Management is not only a matter of leadership, it also involves aptitudes and ability; in simple terms, a manager is one who gets his work done by getting others to do theirs. He must show an intelligent and humane understanding of the needs of the enterprise and of the people who work within the enterprise for him. Good management is about setting goals and objectives and knowing how to achieve them. Like the process of nursing, the process of management involves a number of definable stages of operations:

Planning

Predicting events and deciding in advance how to approach problems.

Deciding on a course of action, that is, what needs to be done, how and when it should be done, and who should do it.

Directing

Creating a favourable working atmosphere and providing positive and direct leadership where necessary.

Coordinating and implementing actions

Ensuring a unity of action towards a commonly accepted goal.

Evaluation

Checking results against the original plan of action and taking corrective measures as they are identified as being required.

Communication

Providing an effective means of allowing a two-way dialogue between the manager and his team.

All of these principles can be applied to all management roles in all settings. Without a clear understanding of these matters, the manager will be blind to the realities of life around him and will provide poor leadership which will result in poor performance.

There have been moves in recent years to base clinical practice in nursing on a problem-solving approach. Hopefully, this philosophy will broaden until its principles are understood and applied in all branches of the profession, that is, in management and in teaching as well as in clinical practice.

Nurses trained on traditional task-orientated models are destined to become purely task-orientated managers. It is exceedingly difficult to undo the learning and conditioning of a lifetime's professional training and work. It is at the stage of nurse training when we have the young student nurse with an open mind that we need to develop the skills which will prepare the nurse for her future role within the profession, be that as a clinical practitioner, as a teacher or as a manager.

Suggested further reading

Anthony, W. (1981) *Management Competencies and Incompetencies*. London: Addison-Wesley.

British Institute of Management: *Code of Conduct and Supporting Guides to Good Management Practice*.

Burns, T. & Stalker, G.M. (1961) *The Management of Innovation*. London: Tavistock Institute for Human Relations.

Forrest, A. (1983) *The Manager's Guide to Setting Targets*. London: Industrial Society.

Glass, P.J. (1971) *Management in a Nutshell*. Available from Filton Technical College, Filton, Bristol.

Haywood, S.C. (1974) *Managing the Health Service*. London: George Allen & Unwin.

MacGregor, D. (1960) *The Human Side of Enterprise*. New York: McGraw Hill.

MacGregor, D. (1967) (ed. C. MacGregor & W. Dennis) *The Professional Manager*. New York: McGraw Hill.

Nolan, V. (1981) *Open to Change*. London: MCB Publications.

Raybould, E. (ed.) (1977) *A Guide for Nurse Managers*. Oxford: Blackwell Scientific Publications.

Schurr, M. (1968) *Leadership and the Nurse*. Sevenoaks: English Universities Press.

Skinner, W. (1981) Big hat—no cattle—managing human resources. *Harvard Business Review*, September/October, pp. 106–114. Available from the British Institute of Management.

Stewart, R. (1979) *The Reality of Management*. London: Pan Books.

Wissema, J. & Van De Winkel, J. (1981) Management in the 80's—how is the job changing? *Long Range Planning*, Vol. 14, No. 4, pp. 21–23. Available from the British Institute of Management.

Chapter 3
Industrial Relations Within the National Health Service

RAY ROWDEN

The subject of industrial relations is about how people interact with one another at work. It is only recently that the National Health Service in general, and nurses in particular, have really come to grips with the need for a systematised industrial relations framework.

Prior to the 1974 National Health Service reorganisation, most health care enterprises were unaware of the subject of industrial relations, and had few rules to facilitate good communications between managers and health workers.

Industrial relations is generally considered to be a complex subject; there are many different theories postulated about it. Some researchers and writers hold the view that relationships between workers and managers are based on a mutually common interest, that is, the successful functioning of any enterprise is good for all. This approach fosters a view that union representatives and managers must work harmoniously together and that this is best achieved by a democratic management style where consensus can be reached by discussion. Others, however, take an opposite view and feel that there are, and always will be, fundamental conflicts of interest within a society based on a capitalist model, and that the interests of capital and labour are bound to clash within industrial relations systems.

Both approaches have some validity. There are many managers and stewards who accept the consensus-common-interest view; equally, there are those who hold the opposing view. In the United Kingdom, the industrial relations framework has generally been biased towards a consensus model where conflicts can be minimised.

Conflict in the work-place, particularly in health care, can be costly and extremely dangerous. It is, therefore, wise to minimise disputes by whatever means possible in the work setting. In traditional industrial settings, the model of industrial relations adopted often appears to be based on the conflict theory.

Within nursing, however, it is much more difficult to identify who is a worker and who is a manager. In nursing, bargaining for salaries and conditions of service is highly centralised at national level and it therefore follows that the decisions made in this arena affect the most senior nurse manager and the most junior nurse in much the same way.

Within this structure there is a great deal of common interest between the manager and the worker. This is witnessed by the fact that many nurses, whether in clinical practice or management, belong to the same unions. This pattern of trade union membership is not so common in other occupational groups within society.

It is perhaps for this reason that nurses in management have generally found a consensus approach to industrial relations to be the most workable and appropriate. However, this does not mean that conflicts never arise or that the nurse manager is never faced with the truculent shop steward stereotype.

Although salaries and conditions of service are settled at a national level, there are still many matters that are settled locally and it is in this area that the nurse manager will be closely involved. Nurses in management need to be familiar with the industrial relations framework pertaining to the National Health Service if they are to play a part in achieving good relationships in the work setting.

The National Health Service is a large multi-professional, multi-craft industry employing millions of people. It therefore follows that the industrial relations systems have to be complex to be able to meet the needs and expectations of all groups within the service. There is a logical structure to the industrial relations framework within the National Health Service and the manager who is familiar with and understands that framework will benefit from this knowledge.

Trade unions are increasing their activity within the nursing profession and many nurses are now undertaking the duties of shop stewardship on behalf of their respective trade unions and organisations. Nearly all trade unions train their local representatives very effectively in industrial relations. If the line manager is to function effectively, he/she must be as well informed as the staff representative he/she meets in the course of his/her work.

It is also important that the manager should be in a position where he/she is able to provide his/her staff with full and adequate information about such matters as salaries and conditions of service.

Many problems arise in nursing because of a lack of understanding about industrial relations within the National Health Service on the part of nurse managers. Some of these problems could be alleviated by a greater understanding of industrial relations systems and bargaining institutions currently operating within the National Health Service. This chapter should assist the reader to gain a greater insight into this important area of management.

TRADE UNIONS AND PROFESSIONAL ORGANISATIONS OPERATING WITHIN NURSING

There are a large number of trade unions involving themselves with nursing. There are over 34 organisations claiming to have nurses in their membership. It is necessary to be familiar with the major organisations involved in nursing and some information about union membership patterns within the workplace can be useful to the manager in deciding who to consult with at local level. The major organisations fall into two main categories:

1. Unions or organisations that have a multi-occupational membership.
2. Those exclusively dealing with nurses, midwives or health visitors.

There is one further difference to consider when dealing with trade union structures. Some unions are affiliated to the Trades Union Congress (TUC) and others are not. In recent years, there has been some confusion over the position and rights of non-TUC-affiliated unions within the National Health Service.

TUC affiliation, in itself, confers no greater rights to a trade union within law. What is important is that any organisation claiming to be a trade union must be registered with the certification officer under the terms and conditions of the Trade Union and Labour Relations Act 1974. All the organisations active within nursing are so registered and enjoy equal privileges and rights within the terms of the Trade Union and Labour Relations Act.

Multi-occupational trade unions

Confederation of Health Service Employees (COHSE)

General Secretary: David Williams, RMN
Headquarters: High Street, Banstead, Surrey SM7 2LH
Telephone: Burgh Heath (073 73) 53322

A specialist trade union catering for all grades of staff within the National Health Service. COHSE claims a large level of nurses in its membership and is particularly active in the psychiatric and mental handicap fields. The union is organised on a local branch basis, the branch secretary being a key local figure to whom local stewards relate. It is represented on the Nurses' and Midwives' Whitley Council. It is affiliated to the Labour Party and the TUC. The union has various regional offices with paid full-time officials.

General and Municipal Workers' Union (GMWU)

General Secretary: David Basnett
Headquarters: Thorne House, Ruxley Ridge, Claygate, Esher, Surrey
Telephone: Esher (0372) 62081

The GMWU is the third largest union in the United Kingdom and is a mass membership general trade union. The union has a non-manual section within its structure, the Managerial, Administrative, Technical and Supervisory Association (MATSA) to which nurses and midwives may belong. The union has a low level of nurse membership, but it does enjoy local pockets of strong activity within nursing. It is organised on a local branch basis, the branch secretary being a key local figure to whom local stewards relate. The union is represented on the Nurses' and Midwives' Whitley Council. It is affiliated to the Labour Party and the TUC. The union has various regional offices with paid full-time officials.

National and Local Government Officers' Association (NALGO)

General Secretary: G.A. Drain, BA, LLB, JP
Headquarters: 1 Mabledon Place, London WC1H GAJ
Telephone: 01-388 2366

NALGO is the fourth largest union in the United Kingdom, representing administrative, clerical, professional and technical staff in the public services. The union claims a large nursing membership, particularly among qualified grades. It is organised on a local district and branch basis, with the branch secretary being a key local figure to whom stewards relate. The union has a health services section and a national officer dealing specifically with health service members and their problems. It is represented on the Nurses' and Midwives' Whitley Council. It is affiliated to the TUC. The union has various regional offices with paid full-time officials.

National Union of Public Employees (NUPE)

General Secretary: Rodney Bickerstaffe
Headquarters: Civic House, Aberdeen Terrace, Blackheath, London SE3 0QY
Telephone: 01-852 2842

NUPE is a large multi-occupational union operating in all areas of the public sector, particularly in ancillary grades. The union is strongly active in most areas of the National Health Service and claims a large nursing membership, particularly among nursing auxiliaries. NUPE has a reputation as being among the more militant trade unions operating within the National Health Service. It is organised on a local branch basis with the branch secretary being a key figure to whom local stewards relate. The union has a health services committee at national level which deals with matters related to its health service members and their problems. It is affiliated to the Labour Party and the TUC. NUPE is represented on the Nurses' and Midwives' Whitley Council. The union has various regional offices with paid full-time officials.

Transport and General Workers' Union (TGWU)

General Secretary: Mostyn Evans
Headquarters: Transport House, Smith Square, London SW1T 3JB
Telephone: 01-828 7788

The TGWU is the largest trade union in the country with approximately two million members. The union has a public services section under which its nurse members are organised. It is mainly active among National Health Service ancillary staff and among nursing auxiliaries. The union is organised on a local branch basis with the branch secretary being a key figure to whom local stewards relate. The TGWU is not represented on the Nurses' and Midwives' Whitley Council. It is affiliated to the Labour Party and the TUC. The union has various regional offices with paid full-time officials.

Specialised unions and professional organisations

Association of Nurse Administrators (ANA)

Hon. Secretary: Maureen Fraser-Gambell, BA, SRN, SCM
Headquarters: 13 Grosvenor Place, London SW1X 7EN
Telephone: 01-235 5258

The ANA is a small specialist organisation with membership limited to nurses registered on the general part of the General Nursing Council register, who are in a management position within the nursing service. The ANA functions as a trade union on behalf of its members through local representatives and is organised on a branch basis with branches related to health authorities. ANA is represented on the Nurses' and Midwives' Whitley Council. The union has no regional offices.

Health Visitors' Association (HVA)

General Secretary: Shirley Goodwin, SRN, HV Cert.
Headquarters: 36 Eccleston Square, London SW1V 1PS
Telephone: 01-834 9523

The HVA is a small specialised organisation specifically for health visitors with an associate membership grade for school nurses. It functions as a trade union with local stewards and also operates as an educational body for health visitors. The HVA is organised into local centres related to health authorities. The HVA is represented on the Nurses' and Midwives' Whitley Council. It is affiliated to the TUC. The union has no regional offices.

Royal College of Midwives (RCM)

General Secretary: Ruth Ashton, SRN, SCM, MTD
Headquarters: 15 Mansfield Street, London W1NM OBE.

The Royal College of Midwives is an educational and professional organisation as well as being an independent trade union. It is exclusively for midwives and pupil midwives. The RCM has a separate labour relations and legal department, with full-time specialist officers who deal with the trade union activity. The RCM provides its members with professional indemnity insurance cover. It is represented on the Nurses' and Midwives' Whitley Council. The RCM has no regional offices.

Royal College of Nursing of the United Kingdom (RCN)

General Secretary: Trevor Clay, SRN, RMN, M.Phil
Headquarters: Cavendish Square, London W1M OAB
Telephone: 01-409 3333

The Rcn is an educational and professional organisation as well as an independent trade union exclusively for nurses holding a statutory qualification or those in training for a statutory qualification. The Rcn has a separate labour relations and legal department with specialised officers and solicitors to deal with the trade union activities of the organisation. The Rcn has a local stewards scheme to provide members with local representation. It provides its members with professional indemnity insurance cover. The Rcn is organised on a local centre basis, usually related to health authorities, and the centres do not normally deal directly with industrial relations matters at local level. The stewards have a local committee structure in most health authorities for the conduct of industrial relations on behalf of its membership. The Rcn is represented on the Nurses' and Midwives' Whitley Council. The Rcn has various regional offices with paid full-time officers.

Scottish Association of Nurse Administrators (SANA)

Hon. Secretary: Miss S. Mitchell
Headquarters: Victoria Infirmary, Langside, Glasgow G42 9TY
Telephone: 041-649 4545

The constitution and role of the Scottish ANA are similar to the constitution and role of its English counterpart.

Scottish Health Visitors' Association (SHVA)

Secretary: Mrs S. Aitken
Headquarters: 12 Niven Road, Inverkeithing, Fife KY11 1Ed
Telephone: 0383 4415149

The constitution and role of the Scottish HVA are similar to those of its English counterpart.

The manager and the trade union representative

Having examined the basic details of the major trade unions, the manager needs to know what to expect of the union representative. Most, if not all, of the major trade unions operating in nursing train their local representatives extremely effectively in industrial relations practice. The manager should bear this in mind.

Relations with local representatives are crucial to the smooth running of any enterprise and it is helpful to understand the role of the union representative. It is wise to take a positive view of the local representative. He has usually been elected by, or enjoys the support of, his colleagues and he deserves respect and courtesy, not only as an employee but as an independent representative of his organisation and its members.

The sensible manager will view the local union representative as a useful agent in effective management. The days of the cloth cap image of the union man in industrial relations circles have largely gone. Modern industrial relations systems are far too complex for the barrack-room-lawyer type to survive for long.

The trade union representative of today will be well versed in all aspects of his job and will probably not tolerate the table-thumping dictatorial manager. To the secure manager, an intelligent, well-versed union representative who is in touch with his members and represents their interests in a responsible manner is a valuable asset. To the insecure, ill-prepared manager, he is an enormous threat.

So what does a union representative's job involve? The union representative has a wide range of duties which will depend greatly on the rules of his own organisation but, in broad terms, the trade union representative has the following responsibilities:

Trade union organisation

Recruiting members
Arranging local publicity for his organisation
Attending meetings of various types involving union work

Handling members' problems

Representing members involved in disciplinary action
Representing members who feel aggrieved at work

National and local negotiations

The interpretation of national agreements from Whitley Councils
Grading problems
Incorrect payment of salaries and wages
Special-duty and on-call payments
Local negotiation of policies and procedures
Local negotiations involving facilities for staff, for example, nurses' residences

Health and safety matters

Accident reports
Safety committees
Hazards and dangers at work

Manpower matters

Overtime working (where appropriate)
Shift system negotiations
Staffing levels
Redundancy and job loss
Early retirement on health grounds
Training of fellow employees

Matters involving employment law

Maternity pay cases
Unfair dismissal
Industrial injuries and compensation claims
Equal opportunities cases

It is easy to see from the above that the trade union representative is entrusted with heavy responsibilities by his organisation and by his members. The manager who approaches his relationships with trade union representatives with empathy and respect will be far more successful than the autocrat who takes the view that a management position gives him the divine right to lay down the law in all matters.

Trade union representatives, like managers, are not always perfect. Some may be poorly trained and some may appear to be very irresponsible. Some will even be rude and aggressive. It is important that the manager faced with this type of representative maintains a calm demeanour. It will not assist any situation if the manager adopts a similar style. Industrial relations in the National Health Service involve a great amount of thought and, above all, patience.

THE NATIONAL HEALTH SERVICE BARGAINING FRAMEWORK

At the time of the establishment of the National Health Service in 1948, it was apparent that salaries and conditions of service within the health care scene were widely variable. In order to streamline this, the government of the day established a national system for determining salaries and conditions of service for staff in the new health service.

This development was thought desirable for a number of reasons. First, the government felt that planning and financing the new National Health Service would become more predictable if all establishments had common salaries and conditions. Unions favoured a national bargaining system since their local organisation at that time was poor.

The model chosen was the Whitley Council system and this method of settling pay and conditions has remained in existence virtually unchanged since its inception. Whitley Councils have a staff side consisting of representatives selected by relevant trade unions and professional organisations and who elect their own staff side officers and a management side drawn from the health authorities, government departments and the civil service. In the light of the establishment of a pay review body for nurses, the management side is likely to be reduced. The Nurses' and Midwives' Whitley Council will in future deal only with conditions of service; the management side will consist mainly of senior civil servants.

The management sides of other functional councils are nominated by health authorities and appointed by the Secretary of State and are provided with a secretariat from senior civil servants within the Department of Health and Social Security.

In basic terms, the staff side and the management side meet together on a regular basis and discuss and negotiate salaries and conditions of service pertinent to their staff group. The management side frequently has to return to ministers and civil servants for guidance in the bargaining process and the unions frequently have to return to their members for guidance.

Bargaining for salaries and conditions within this framework can be extremely slow and, at times, cumbersome. The system has, however, worked reasonably well to date. There are in all ten functional Whitley Councils representing various grades and types of staff within the National Health Service. They are:

Administrative and Clerical Whitley Council
Ambulancemen's Whitley Council
Ancillary Staffs' Whitley Council
Medical and (Hospital) Dental Whitley Council
Nurses' and Midwives' Whitley Council
Optical Staffs' Whitley Council
Pharmaceutical Staffs' Whitley Council

Professional and Technical Staffs A Whitley Council
Professional and Technical Staffs B Whitley Council
Dental (Local Authorities) Whitley Council

The Nurses' and Midwives' Whitley Council is made up of the following representatives:

Management side

	Members
Regional Health Authorities	5
English Health Authorities	6
Scottish Health Authorities	3
Welsh Health Authorities	1
Department of Health and Social Security	3
Scottish Home and Health Department	1
Welsh Office	1

This structure will change in the near future, with greater representation from the government departments.

Staff side

	Members
Association of Nurse Administrators	1
Association of Hospital and Residential Care Officers	1
Association of Supervisors of Midwives	1
Confederation of Health Service Employees	4
Health Visitors' Association	2
Managerial, Administrative, Technical and Supervisory Association	1
National and Local Government Officers' Association	2
National Union of Public Employees	4
Royal College of Midwives	3
Royal College of Nursing	8
Scottish Association of Nurse Administrators	1
Scottish Health Visitors' Association	1

Following the establishment of the Pay Review Body, the government has suggested a reduction in the size of the staff side. In Northern Ireland there is an independent Whitley Council system in operation: this, too, will be changed in structure and function by the newly established Pay Review Body.

With members and civil service support, the Nurses' and Midwives' Whitley Council has nearly 50 members. It would be extremely difficult, if not impossible, to conduct delicate negotiations in a group of this size. To overcome this problem, the Nurses' and Midwives' Whitley Council has a smaller negotiating committee which actually sits around the table to reach agreements. Both sides of this committee have to continually refer back to the full council for guidance during negotiations.

Prior to 1983 all agreements on salaries and specific conditions for nurses and midwives were reached through this machinery. Following the establishment of the Pay Review Body, only nurses' and midwives' conditions of service will be dealt with in this way. Agreements on all matters are laid out in writing in the form of an advanced letter to health authorities which authorises the implementation of an agreement at local level.

The text of the advanced letter then becomes part of the Whitley Council handbook. It can be easily seen that a word out of place in such an agreement can have enormous ramifications throughout the service. For this reason, the wording of all advanced letters has to be agreed between both sides of the council prior to implementation.

This process can be extremely complicated and because of this, delays can sometimes occur between the reaching of an agreement and its implementation at local level. Within this highly centralised bargaining system there is a great deal of ambiguity in the interpretation of Whitley Council rules and regulations.

To deal with such ambiguity, the Whitley Council has a structured system of appeals for clarification of agreements. This machinery is explained in section XXII of the General Whitley Council conditions of service handbook. This process begins at the local level and a matter of dispute can be taken through various levels up to the full national Whitley Council if interpretation cannot be agreed upon.

THE PAY REVIEW MACHINERY

The Whitley Council ceased to negotiate salaries for nurses and midwives following the establishment of the Pay Review Body. This consists of an independent chairman and seven members from outside the service.

This machinery will also be used to determine levels of remuneration for other groups of para-medical staff, for example, radiographers, physiotherapists and occupational therapists. In simple terms, the review body will invite interested parties to submit evidence related to earnings. The trade unions and the Department of Health will be involved in this process. The review body will have civil service support and access to a wide range of data related to earnings in all sectors of the economy.

When the review body has examined all evidence, it will report directly to the government of the day, recommending salary levels. The government may or may not accept the report of the review body. It is after this stage that a pay award is sanctioned by the Secretary of State and authority given to make payment.

WHAT WILL THE NURSES' AND MIDWIVES' WHITLEY COUNCIL DO?

The organisations represented on the staff side of the Nurses' and Midwives' Whitley Council will continue to act in unison when preparing and submitting evidence to the review body whenever possible. It might weaken the validity of evidence if each union goes its own way in submitting views to the review body. In this area the staff side will have a great deal of work to undertake collectively. Equally, the management side, representing the interests of the DOHSS and health authorities, will want to reach common agreement in relation to submission of evidence. Although we can expect to see a smaller functional council for nurses and midwives, it is evident that their actual function will not alter too radically in the light of the pay review machinery.

In addition to salaries, the council will still need to negotiate issues related to conditions of service for nurses and midwives and will continue to have an active interest in generic issues raised at the General Whitley Council. The doctors and dentists have had a review mechanism for many years; they still retain a functional Whitley Council to deal with conditions of service and retain an active interest in the affairs of the general council.

THE GENERAL WHITLEY COUNCIL FOR THE HEALTH SERVICES

The General Whitley Council's function is to negotiate certain conditions of service, not salaries, pertinent to all the functional councils. Matters such as travelling and removal expenses, arrangements for redundancy payments and assistance with house purchase are all examples of matters dealt with by this council. The council is made up of the following representatives:

Management side

	Members
Department of Health and Social Security	3
Scottish Home and Health Department	1
Welsh Office	1
Regional Health Authorities	6
English Health Authorities	7
Scottish Health Authorities	5
Welsh Health Authorities	3

Staff side

	Members
Administrative and Clerical Whitley Council	4
Ambulancemen's Whitley Council	2
Ancillary Staffs' Whitley Council	4
Medical and (Hospital) Dental Whitley Council	4
Nurses' and Midwives' Whitley Council	4
Optical Staffs' Whitley Council	1
Pharmaceutical Staffs' Whitley Council	3
Professional and Technical Staffs A Whitley Council	3
Professional and Technical Staffs B Whitley Council	3
Dental (Local Authorities) Whitley Council	1

The representatives on the staff side of the General Whitley Council are chosen by their respective functional councils.

The manager will find all information related to salaries and conditions of service within the handbooks issued by the Nurses' and Midwives' Whitley Council and the General Whitley Council for Health Services.

It is useful for the manager to have easy access to both handbooks. Agreements reached at national level are frequently subject to much local discussion as to interpretation. The manager should be familiar with the Whitley regulations and time taken to study new national agreements is time well spent.

Mistakes in payments and conditions of service can be costly and can create a great deal of ill-feeling between management and staff at local level.

The manager who has taken time to familiarise himself/herself with the Whitley Council regulations can minimise the chance of mistakes occurring. Copies of the Whitley Council's handbooks can be obtained for a small charge from the following addresses:

The General Whitley Council Handbook

Management Side Secretary
General Whitley Council for the Health Services (Great Britain)
Friars House
157/168 Blackfriars Road
London SE1 8EU

Nurses' and Midwives' Whitley Council Handbook

Management Side Secretary
Nurses' and Midwives' Whitley Council
Hannibal House
Elephant and Castle
London SE1 6TE

LOCAL CONSULTATIVE MACHINERY

The General Whitley Council has recommended that joint consultative committees consisting of management and staff representatives should be established at all hospitals and community units within the service. The majority of health authorities within the United Kingdom have some form of established joint consultative machinery. The functions of the local joint consultative committee are outlined in section XXIV of the General Whitley Council handbook are are defined as follows:

(a) To promote the closest cooperation and provide a recognised means of consultation between the health authority, its senior officers and staff.
(b) To give the staffs a wider interest in and a greater responsibility for the conditions under which their work is performed to give the maximum assistance in promoting the welfare of the patients and efficient administration in the hospitals controlled by the authority. To make suggestions for the improvement of the general arrangements for the comfort of the staff, their recreation, entertainment and diet.

(c) To prevent friction and misunderstanding.
(d) Subject to the provisos that no recommendations of the local staffs committee shall conflict with, or override, any decision of the General Council or the appropriate functional council, to deal with such matters as: (i) the distribution of working hours, (ii) holiday arrangements, (iii) questions of physical welfare, e.g., cloakroom arrangements, heating and ventilation, etc.
(e) To consider any hospital rules affecting staff apart from any that may be prescribed nationally or regionally.

The constitution of the local joint consultative committee as recommended by the General Whitley Council has provided for staff representatives to be elected on an occupational group basis, that is, administrative and clerical representatives, nurses' and midwives' representatives, domestic, farm and garden staff representatives, etc.

The rules of the constitution have stipulated that staff representatives so elected must be members of a trade union or professional organisation represented on a functional Whitley Council. Many health authorities operate their joint consultative machinery on this model, but in recent years many health authorities have allowed joint consultative committees to allocate staff side seats on a recognised trade union or professional organisation basis, that is, Rcn representative, NUPE representative, COHSE representative, etc.

Many trade unions and organisations within the National Health Service favour the latter approach to the formation of joint consultative committees. Membership of the management side of joint consultative committees is decided by the local management team, but will always include a nurse member. Joint consultative committees operate at varying levels within the health service and some health authorities may have one overall committee to discuss all matters pertinent to staff within the employ of the authority. Others may have more locally based joint consultative committees related to individual hospitals or community units.

Joint consultative machinery has often been criticised by trade unions within the health service as being nothing more than 'talk shops', with little real value. It is important that consultation is seen to be meaningful and effective if it is to function successfully at the local level.

Management should not always arrive at meetings to consult on a matter that is already a *fait accompli*, but should seek to allow staff maximum genuine participation in the decision-making processes of the enterprise. Failure to operate effective joint consultative machinery can often lead to a sense of frustration and mistrust in staff representatives, who, when consultative machinery fails them, will be put into a position where they have to formally involve their trade union in a dispute situation.

Well-managed effective joint consultative committees can prevent a deterioration in industrial relations at local level and the nurse manager involved in such a committee should take a full and active part in the activities of the joint consultative committee.

NEGOTIATING WITH RECOGNISED TRADE UNIONS

Many matters of importance to the conduct of industrial relations cannot be dealt with in the joint consultative committee model. With the increasing influence of employment legislation, and of trade unionism within the National Health Service, the list of matters likely to require formal negotiation with trade unions is likely to grow.

In order to establish a forum for formal discussion of such matters, many areas of the health service are establishing joint union committees. Some areas have committees consisting of senior representatives from all health service organisations represented on functional Whitley Councils. Other areas have established committees for TUC-affiliated unions with separate machinery for the non-TUC-affiliates.

These committees will normally meet management formally on a regular basis to discuss such matters as disciplinary procedures, grievance procedures, redundancy policies, policies for reallocation of staff, facilities for union representatives, etc.

The representatives on this type of committee will usually be experienced senior stewards or branch secretaries, and it is in this arena that much formal bargaining and negotiation occurs. There is no nationally agreed constitution for such committees and their recognition or non-recognition will be dependent upon the policy of individual local health authorities.

THE BARGAINING PROCESS

In dealing with local negotiations, it is wise to understand what is involved in the bargaining and negotiating process. When managers and unions meet formally in whatever setting, they will rightly have different viewpoints and objectives related to the matter under discussion.

Industrial relations is about reaching the most effective compromise, where conflicting interests can be minimised to produce mutually satisfactory agreement. This process involves a great deal of psychology and the nurse has many basic skills that can be utilised in his/her role as a manager in this setting.

Within the health service, the number and complexity of different bargaining situations is enormous, but the following rules can be applied to almost all situations where formal bargaining and negotiation is involved.

There is a fundamental difference between joint consultative and collective bargaining at local level. The consultative model within the National Health Service usually operates on the basis that management reserves the right to take decisions after consultation even if the union representatives disagree. In genuine collective bargaining situations, particularly with joint trade union committees, either side cannot proceed without agreement on the subject under discussion. In the formation of policies related to the conduct of industrial relations, it is widely accepted that agreement between management and unions is vital if such policies are to be effectively implemented.

Some useful guidelines

The first, and some would say, most important step in any effective negotiating process is in the preparation of the case under discussion. It is important that the manager is clear about his/her objective for meeting with unions.

Prior to meeting, the manager should identify clearly the goal of the meeting. It is also sensible to establish a fall-back position, that is, the lowest settlement that is acceptable to management. Factual information is always a vital element in any situation involving negotiating, and the manager should collect relevant factual data and arrange it in a clear, concise and logical form for use and presentation.

It is helpful to make a written itemised list of points prior to any meeting, placing the most important items the manager wishes to raise uppermost on the list. This can be helpful as an *aide-mémoire* and can also ensure that points are not overlooked in heated debate.

Empathy is a skill associated with nursing; it also has validity in industrial relations. The manager should always attempt to analyse the union position; this can help to prevent intransigence on the part of the manager. It can also help the manager to gain a deeper understanding of what is making the union representative tick.

Intelligent forethought will also focus the mind on the strong and weak points of the other side's case and one can think more objectively about one's responses to that case. Having prepared and documented a case, the manager should be clear prior to any meeting who is to present the management case.

On many occasions, formal negotiation will occur with a management team. It is important that each member of that team understands his part in the presentation of the case. Where the nurse manager is to be one member of the team, it is helpful to have a pre-meeting meeting to discuss these matters in detail. If managers are ill-prepared for negotiation, a situation could arise where decisions are made which are unacceptable to individual managers. It is too late to complain in the middle of a delicate discussion with union representatives.

THE BARGAINING SETTING

It is when the manager actually sits at the negotiating table that the psychology of bargaining becomes useful and applicable. The following points are well worth bearing in mind.

First, plan the layout of the room carefully and sit where you feel most comfortable. It is a matter of choice, but it may be preferable for you sometimes to take the seat at the head of the table; in other settings, it may be wise to take a less dominant position. It may also on occasions be useful to have a very informal setting with perhaps a circle of chairs around a low table. Think carefully about the purpose of the meeting, who you are meeting and plan the environment accordingly.

Keen observation of human behaviour is another nursing skill that has valid application in industrial relations. Where, for instance, does the union representative position himself in a bargaining situation? If a group is to be met, do they all sit together? Do they split and mingle with management representatives? Does the individual present a calm and relaxed picture or is he fidgeting with the pen in his hand or the ring on his finger? Will he avoid eyeball-to-eyeball contact during discussion or does he appear comfortable and confident in the situation?

All of these observations of non-verbal cues can tell the manager a great deal about the way in which the union representative views his case. Again, empathy is important in actual face-to-face discussions. Total intransigence is not a useful posture to adopt. During the meeting the manager should keep uppermost in his/her mind the objectives of management.

Careful listening is also vital, for offers from union representatives may be phrased in a guarded way. If so, it will be necessary to clarify exactly what compromise is possible and the terms of that compromise.

Use adjournments wisely in negotiations. It may be necessary to break off discussions in order for management to review their position behind closed doors.

Discussion should stick to the point. Rambling debate that shoots off in all directions is not helpful to achieving a satisfactory solution and is also a waste of valuable time. It is often salutary to cost particular meetings. If one begins to consider the hourly rate of pay of managers and employee representatives in meetings, one begins to realise that time, even in the National Health Service, is money!

One vital point to remember is never allow discussion to deteriorate into a slanging match. To lose control of one's temper in a discussion of this nature is a great failure, and self-control, even if one feels extremely provoked, is vital. It is sometimes the case that a union representative may actually attempt to bring about this situation. The wise manager will learn never to take things too personally in the industrial relations game; that is the way to prevent this deterioration from occurring.

Equally, it is never acceptable for the manager to become rude or abusive in dealings with staff representatives in formalised bargaining settings.

In discussions that involve the application of particular rules or procedures, for example, a Whitley Council agreement governing the matter under consideration, or a local or disciplinary or grievance procedure, it is essential that the manager be totally familiar with the relevant documentary background and keep copies close at hand for immediate reference during meetings. Failure to strictly observe any rules that are laid down can lead to managers losing a case and if, for example, a disciplinary matter is misjudged and subsequently goes to tribunal, this can cost the employer a great deal of money. The manager who is conversant with any relevant written rules or procedures will also be in a position to ensure that the union representatives are playing the game according to the rules.

Having reached an agreement, it is necessary and important that the terms of agreement be set out in writing. This is in everybody's interests and may prevent misunderstanding at a later stage. Most unions advise their representatives not to leave a bargaining situation without seeing written terms of agreement.

In many cases, this will not always be possible, and the manager should always be prepared to meet again to draft agreements for joint consideration. It is, however, advisable to commit agreements to paper as quickly as possible, while the nature of the debate is fresh in the mind.

While industrial relations is a complex subject, it is also fascinating, involving the application of forethought and intelligence. The rewards for the manager of skilled industrial relations practice are high. Disruption in the work-place and the subsequent ill-feeling that such disruption invariably creates is well worth avoiding.

The manager who is equipped to approach industrial relations with confidence will often succeed in minimising conflicts at work. The manager who takes no time to study industrial relations and who manages entirely by gut reaction and guess-work is destined, sooner or later, to abject failure in this vital aspect of management.

Suggested further reading

Barrett, B., Rhodes, E. & Beishon, J. (eds) (1975) *Industrial Relations and the Wider Society—Aspects of Interaction*. Milton Keynes: Open University Press.

Davies, C. (ed.) (1980) *Re-writing Nursing History*. London: Croom Helm. (See in particular Chapter 7, The History of the Present Contradiction and Struggle in Nursing, by Paul Bellaby and Patric Oribabor.)

Dunlop, J.T. (1958) *Industrial Relations Systems*. New York: Holt, Rinehart and Winston.

Flanders, A. (1970) *Management and Unions*. London: Faber & Faber.

Making Whitley Work (1976) Report of Lord McCarthy on the Whitley Council within the National Health Service. London: HMSO.

Rowden, R. (1977) The complete steward. *Nursing Standard* (RCN), October.

The General Whitley Council for the Health Services (Great Britain) Handbook.

The Nurses' and Midwives' Whitley Council Handbook.

TUC (1975) *Good Industrial Relations: TUC Guide for Negotiators.*

Chapter 4
Employment Law and Industrial Relations Legislation

RAY ROWDEN

The law concerning the regulation of relationships between employers and employees is complex and continually changing. Employment law mushroomed during the 1970s and continues to develop. The nurse manager need not have an encyclopaedic knowledge of all legislation, but it is advisable and, indeed, practically useful to have a broad insight into the effects of the major pieces of legislation relating to this subject.

This chapter should assist the reader in gaining a basic knowledge of the subject and should guide the reader to further, more detailed information where this is required. It has to be recognised that all major trade unions attempt to provide their work-place representatives with a basic understanding of employment legislation; it therefore follows that the manager must be similarly apprised if he is to function effectively.

GENERAL SOURCES OF INFORMATION

The body of law relating to employment is constantly changing and it is not always possible to be completely up-to-date with all the nuances of the law. There are, however, some simple steps that any manager can take to keep his knowledge reasonably updated.

1. Many government departments and agencies such as the Department of Employment, the Advisory Conciliation and Arbitration Service, the Health and Safety Commission, the Department of Health and Social Security, the Equal Opportunities Commission, etc. issue excellent leaflets giving sound guidance related to the various pieces of legislation and associated regulations. The government departments routinely update this kind of information and their publications are provided either free of charge or for a very small fee.

2. Many publishing houses have produced reference books for employers which are continually and automatically updated. This service is valuable and costs are reasonable. The subscriber usually pays an initial fee for a loose-leaf bound reference book, followed by an annual subscription. As new law is enacted or existing law altered, the publishers send subscribers update sheets to add to the reference manual. It is highly likely that your health authority personnel department subscribes to a service of this kind.
3. The more serious daily newspapers frequently publish law reviews relating to industrial relations legislation. Major cases involving employment appeal tribunals, etc. are excellently covered in this way. A newspaper report of a major development can often be the quickest method of gaining fresh knowledge related to new developments in this field. *The Times*, *Daily Telegraph* and the *Guardian* devote attention to this subject and can be recommended.

ACTS OF PARLIAMENT REGULATING INDUSTRIAL RELATIONS

Employment Protection Act 1975

This act was designed to improve industrial relations by encouraging the development and strengthening of collective bargaining. It established certain machinery for promoting the improvement of industrial relations in the United Kingdom.

Advisory, Conciliation and Arbitration Service (ACAS)

ACAS is a statutory body established under the Employment Protection Act and its powers and duties include:

1. Offering conciliation and other assistance to help settle any trade dispute.
2. Providing conciliation officers to promote the settlement of complaints made to industrial tribunals.
3. Referring matters in dispute to arbitration or to the central arbitration committee (CAC).
4. Offering advice to employers, employers' associations, workers and trade unions on industrial relations and employment policies and publishing general advice.
5. Enquiring into any question relating to industrial relations in any particular industry or undertaking.

6. Issuing codes of practice containing practical guidance for the promotion of good industrial relations including specific codes.

The certification officer

A certification officer has been appointed by the Secretary of State to control the regulation and registration of trade unions. Any union can apply to the certification officer for a certificate of independence which will give it certain rights and privileges under employment law.

The certification officer has power to make enquiries and to consider any information submitted to him before he decides to issue a certificate to a trade union. He also has the power to withdraw a certificate from a union if he considers that it is no longer an independent organisation. The certification officer has to receive from certificated unions annual returns, rules and other documents related to the trade union. These documents are available for public inspection.

Trade union recognition

Recognition in relation to a trade union means the recognition of the union by an employer or two or more associated employers to any extent for the purposes of collective bargaining. A recognition issue means an issue arising from a request by a trade union for recognition by an employer or two or more associated employers, including, where recognition is already accorded to some extent, a request for further recognition.

An employer does not have to recognise any trade union; however, unions have the right to refer recognition issues directly to ACAS who can investigate and make rulings on the issue.

If ACAS cannot conciliate between the parties then the aggrieved trade union can apply to a central arbitration committee who are empowered to make awards relating to the union's claims where judgement is made in the union's favour.

Disclosure of information

Under the Employment Protection Act, it is the duty of an employer to disclose to representatives of recognised trade unions, on request, all such information relating to his undertaking which is in his possession and is both:

1. information without which the trade union representatives would be to a

material extent impeded in carrying on with the employer collective bargaining and,

2. information which it would be in accordance with good industrial relations practice that he should disclose to them for the purposes of collective bargaining.

ACAS has issued a code of practice determining what would be in accordance with good industrial relations practice. This code of practice gives some examples of information relating to business undertakings which could be relevant in certain collective bargaining situations and some examples are given below:

1. *Pay and benefits*. Principles and structure of payment systems, job evaluation systems and grading criteria, earnings and hours analysed according to work-group, grade, plant, sex, etc. Giving, where appropriate, distributions and make-up of pay showing any additions to basic rate or salary, total pay bill, details of fringe benefits and non-wage labour costs.
2. *Conditions of service*. Policies on recruitment, redeployment, redundancy, training, equal opportunities and promotion, appraisal systems, health, welfare and safety matters.
3. *Manpower*. Numbers employed analysed according to grade, department, location, age and sex. Labour turnover, absenteeism, overtime and short-time working, manning standards, planned changes in work methods, materials, equipment or organisation, available manpower plans, investment plans.
4. *Performance*. Productivity and efficiency data, savings from increased productivity and output, return on capital invested, sales and state of order books.
5. *Financial*. Cost structures, gross and nett profits, sources of earnings, assets, liabilities, allocation of profits, details of government financial assistance, transfer prices, loans to parent or subsidiary companies and interest charged.

These examples are not intended to represent a check list of information that should be provided for all negotiations. Nor are they meant to be an exhaustive list of types of information, as other items may be relevant in particular negotiations.

It can be seen from this short piece of the code of practice that recognised trade unions do, indeed, have a right in law to an enormous amount of information.

If a local management team is making decisions about the number of nurses employed in a particular area, the local trade union representative can ask for a great deal of information related to such an issue and it is clear that the nurse manager must be prepared to think about what information can and cannot be disclosed to representatives.

The code stresses that employers should aim to be as open and as helpful as possible in meeting trade union requests for information. Where a request for information is refused, the reasons for refusal should be explained as far as possible to the trade union concerned and this should be capable of being substantiated should the matter be taken to the central arbitration committee.

ACAS recommends that employers and trade unions should endeavour to arrive at a joint understanding on how provisions relating to disclosure of information can be implemented most effectively at local level. They should jointly consider what information is likely to be required and what also is available and could be reasonably made available. Consideration should also be given to the form in which the information will be presented, when it should be presented and to whom.

There are certain restrictions on the general duty to disclose information, and these are as follows:

An employer need not disclose:
1. information that is against the interests of national security;
2. information the employer could not disclose without contravening a prohibition imposed under an enactment;
3. information acquired in confidence;
4. information relating specifically to an individual unless he has consented to its disclosure;
5. information likely to cause substantial injury to the employee's/employer's undertaking for reasons other than its effect on collective bargaining;
6. information obtained by the employer for the purpose of bringing, prosecuting or defending any legal proceedings.

Trade Unions and Labour Relations Act 1974

This act sets out to define trade unions' and employers' associations. The act defines a *trade union* as an organisation which either:

1. consists wholly or mainly of workers of one or more descriptions and is an organisation whose principal purposes include the regulation of relations

between workers of that description or those descriptions and employers or employers' associations; or

2. consists wholly or mainly of:
   (a) constituent or affiliated organisations which fulfil those conditions, or
   (b) representatives of such constituent or affiliated organisations and, in either case, is an organisation whose principal purposes include the regulation of relations between workers and employers or between workers' and employers' associations, or include the regulation of relations between its constituent or affiliated organisations.

The act defines an *employers' association* as an organisation which either:

1. consists wholly or mainly of employers or individual proprietors of one or more descriptions and is an organisation whose principal purposes include the regulation of relations between employers of that description or those descriptions and workers or trade unions; or
2. consists wholly or mainly of:
   (a) constituent or affiliated organisations which fulfil the conditions specified in paragraph 1. above, or themselves consist wholly or mainly of constituent or affiliated organisations which fulfil those conditions, or
   (b) representatives of such constituent or affiliated organisations and, in either case, is an organisation whose principal purposes include the regulation of relations between employers and workers, or between employers and trade unions or include the regulation of relations between its constituent or affiliated organisations.

Trade disputes

The Trade Union and Labour Relations Act defines a trade dispute as a dispute between employers and workers or between workers and workers which concerns one of the following:

1. Terms and conditions of employment or the physical conditions in which any workers are required to work.
2. Engagement or non-engagement or termination or suspension of employment or the duties of employment of one or more workers.
3. Allocation of work or the duties of employment as between workers or groups of workers.
4. Matters of discipline.
5. Membership or non-membership of a trade union on the part of a worker.

6. Facilities for officials of trade unions.
7. Machinery for negotiation or consultation and other procedures relating to any of the foregoing matters including the recognition by employers or employers' associations of the right of a trade union to represent workers in any such negotiation or consultation or in the carrying-out of such procedures.

The act also made peaceful picketing other than at a person's residence lawful when carried out in contemplation of furtherance of a trade dispute.

Employment Act 1980

The major effect of this act was to amend previous legislation relating to the conduct of ballots for major decision-making in the trade union movement. The act allows the certification officer to make payments to independent trade unions towards expenditure incurred by them in holding ballots for the following purposes:

1. Obtaining a decision or ascertaining the views of their members on calling or ending strike action.
2. Carrying out elections in accordance with their rules.
3. Amending their rules.
4. Obtaining decisions on amalgamation with other unions or transfer of membership to other unions.
5. Obtaining a decision or ascertaining the views of members as to the acceptance or rejection of an employer's proposal in relation to their contractual terms and conditions of employment.
6. Other matters specified by the Secretary of State.

Employer's premises

If a trade union which is recognised by the employer proposes to hold a ballot for one of the purposes listed above, it has the right to request the employer to allow his premises to be used for the ballot.

A union which is refused permission to do this may complain to an industrial tribunal and awards of compensation may be made where the tribunal finds that the employer's action has been unreasonable.

The Employment Act also allows the Secretary of State to issue codes of practice as he thinks fit for the purpose of improving industrial relations. After consulting with ACAS, a draft of the code must be published and any representations made taken into account. The code must then be approved by the resolution of each House of Parliament before taking effect.

Codes approved under this act include those related to closed shop agreements and arrangements for picketing at the work-place. The power given to the Secretary of State under this act does not in any way take away the power of ACAS to issue its own codes of practice.

Picketing

The act also established regulations defining and controlling the picketing of premises during an industrial dispute. The act outlawed secondary picketing and set limits on the number of pickets allowed.

Employment Protection (Consolidation) Act 1978

This act brought together in one enactment the provisions on individual employment rights previously contained in the following:

Redundancy Payments Act 1965
Contracts of Employment Act 1972
Trade Union and Labour Relations Acts of 1974 and 1976
Employment Protection Act 1975

The Department of Employment publishes a complete list of books and leaflets giving guidance on current employment legislation. Some of the subjects covered are outlined below.

Written statement of main terms and conditions of employment

All employees working 16 hours or more a week must, no later than 13 weeks after employment began, be given either:

1. a written statement giving details of the major conditions of employment; or
2. a written contract of employment which at least incorporates the same details.

The difference between the two is that the second option is actually a contract in writing whereas the first is simply a statement in writing for information purposes, only telling the employee details of the more important terms of employment.

Every statement or contract must:

1. identify the parties to the contract or statement;
2. specify a commencement date;
3. state whether any employment with a previous employer counts as part of the employee's period of continuous employment.

If the employment is for a fixed term only, the expiry date of the contract must also be given. The contract or statement must also itemise the rate of pay or the way pay is worked out and the pay period, that is, hourly/weekly/monthly, etc. as well as:

- any rules as to hours of work including normal working hours
- entitlement to holidays including public holidays and rates of holiday pay
- rules on sickness or injury, absence and sick pay
- details of pension or pension scheme and whether the employee's employment is contracted out of the state pension scheme
- the length of notice the employee is entitled to receive and must give to the employer
- the employee's job title

In addition to the contract or statement, the employee is also entitled to receive copies of any disciplinary rules affecting the employee, plus details of whom the employee can apply to if he is dissatisfied with any disciplinary action taken against him. It is also advisable that a new employee should be given a copy of any relevant grievance procedure with his contract of employment or statement.

Reference documents

As an alternative to an individual contract or statement of employment to each employee, a master document can be used, to which each employee can refer.

If this method is used, written notification has to be given to an employee saying which particulars are contained in the reference document and where the document can be seen. Changes to written particulars listed in a contract or statement of employment must be notified in writing to employees within one month of the change.

Employment rights for the expectant mother

An employee who becomes pregnant may acquire four important rights, which are:

1. not to be unreasonably refused time off for ante-natal care and to be paid when permitted that time off;
2. the right to complain against unfair dismissal because of pregnancy to an industrial tribunal;
3. the right to receive maternity pay;
4. the right to return to work with her employer after a period of absence on account of pregnancy or confinement.

The rights given to pregnant women under the Employment Protection (Consolidation) Act are generally not as favourable as those pertaining to the National Health Service maternity scheme, but can give invaluable protection to nurses employed outside the National Health Service.

Disputes concerning the application of rights under this act can be referred to industrial tribunal. A copy of the National Health Service agreement on maternity leave for employees negotiated by the General Whitley Council can be found in Section VI of the General Council Handbook.

Procedure for handling redundancies

The Employment Protection (Consolidation) Act lays down rules governing the position of the employer and employee in situations where redundancy occurs. Some health authorities have negotiated their own local agreements which go further than the basic rights in law and it is desirable that the manager should be familiar with any local agreement.

The act also details rights of employees given notice of dismissal because of redundancy. Such employees are entitled to reasonable time off work with pay during working hours to look for another job or to make arrangements for training for future employment. Rights under these provisions can be subject to reference to an industrial tribunal.

Dismissal

The act lays down regulations related to the dismissal of employees. The act states that in cases of gross misconduct an employee may be summarily dismissed, that is, dismissed without notice or pay in lieu of notice.

To justify summary dismissal the misconduct must be so serious that it compromises the contract of employment agreed between the employee and employer and the conduct must be such that no reasonable employer could tolerate the continued employment of the employee. Many health authorities are defining quite clearly examples of gross misconduct in disciplinary procedures. It is difficult to produce an exhaustive list of what constitutes gross misconduct, but it is advisable to have some examples established in an agreed procedure.

Defining 'gross misconduct' presents the manager with many problems, for what might constitute gross misconduct in the nursing service need not necessarily apply to other departments within the service. For example, two kitchen workers fighting in a catering area may be given a serious warning regarding their conduct; on the other hand, two nurses fighting physically in the middle of a ward in front of patients would probably be viewed very differently and this might well be taken to constitute gross misconduct.

The act states that any employee with 26 weeks' continuous service is entitled to request a written statement giving a detailed account of the reasons for dismissal:

1. if he is given notice of termination of contract of employment by his employer; or
2. if his contract of employment is terminated without notice by his employer; or
3. where he is employed under a contract for a fixed term and that term expires without being renewed under the same contract.

The employee has a right to this statement within 14 days of the request being made. Unreasonable refusal to give a written statement or a statement that is inaccurate can result in an industrial tribunal awarding two weeks' pay as compensation. The statement provided by the employer is admissible as evidence in any proceedings.

Any worker who has been continuously employed and works for more than 16 hours per week for 52 weeks or more, or who has worked eight hours or more but less than 16 hours a week for a period of five years or more, has the right not to be unfairly dismissed by his employer, and if he is dismissed he has the right to take his case to an industrial tribunal.

There are certain circumstances where this provision does not apply. For example, it does not apply to any employee who before the effective date of termination of employment had reached the age of 65 for men or 60 for women, or the normal retiring age defined by the health authority if this is higher than the normal statutory age limits. The provision also does not apply to employees working under fixed term contracts of one year or more who have agreed in writing to exclude any claim for unfair dismissal and who clearly understand that employment will cease on completion of the fixed term of employment.

The act also lays down very strict rules relating to the dismissal of union officials who feel they are being unfairly treated because of their trade union activities. It is advisable to seek the advice of a senior union official before proceeding with any dismissal proceedings against a local official.

The act also lays down regulations relating to union membership agreements (the closed shop). Dismissal of an employee for refusing to become a member of a specified union where a closed shop exists will be fair if a union membership agreement which covers that employee is in operation. An employee is allowed not to join a union where a closed shop operates if the employee genuinely objects on the grounds of conscience or other deeply held personal conviction to being a member of a trade union. The provisions on closed shop arrangements are currently under close review by the government and it is highly likely that there will be changes in the regulations in the near future.

Dismissal of a pregnant employee. The act states that dismissal of any employee solely because she is pregnant or for any reason connected with her pregnancy will be treated as unfair dismissal, unless because of her pregnancy she is unable adequately to fulfil the terms and conditions of her contract of employment. The employer must offer her suitable alternative work if a vacancy exists in these circumstances. If, however, a vacancy of this nature does not exist, she may be fairly dismissed.

Constructive dismissal. The employment protection act makes it illegal for a manager to put subtle pressure on an employee to cause him to resign from employment. It is exceedingly dangerous to use this method of operation where a manager wishes to get rid of a staff member.

Even where an employee has been persuaded to put his notice in writing to the manager, if subsequently that employee feels that the pressure put on him to resign was unfair, he does have the right to make a claim for constructive dismissal to an industrial tribunal.

Remedies for unfair dismissal. Employees who feel they are unfairly dismissed can choose one of two remedies following successful application to an industrial tribunal. They are entitled either to their job back or to financial recompense.

The tribunal must always approach the remedy first by considering reinstatement or re-engagement and only where this is not possible, or the employee does not choose this option, should they award compensation.

The aim of the tribunal is to restore the worker as nearly as possible to his position before the dismissal. Financial awards are particularly expensive; it is, therefore, advisable to ensure that your authority has strict and clearly understood procedures for the handling of dismissal.

Discipline and dismissal issues are becoming increasingly complicated and advice from the senior nurse personnel should usually be sought when the line manager becomes involved in these issues.

Race Relations Act 1976

This act replaced the Race Relations Acts of 1965 and 1968 and modified and extended the anti-discrimination law provided by them. The act states that job applicants and employees discriminated against can obtain up to £7,000 compensation for loss of employment from an industrial tribunal.

The act abolished a rule which allowed employers to discriminate in order to keep a balance of races among employees; this is no longer allowed. Shop stewards and others acting on behalf of a trade union are no longer personally liable if they discriminate against union applicants or members.

The act also established a commission for racial equality, responsible for policing the provisions of the act and giving guidance related to the working of the act.

Permitted discrimination

The act allows race discrimination in certain very limited circumstances. These provisions are not likely to apply to the nursing service; it is, therefore, quite clear that there is no permitted discrimination for nurse managers.

Unlawful discrimination

The act gives a definition of what amounts to discrimination and goes on to give various examples of activities which employers must not discriminate in doing. Discrimination occurs when, on racial grounds:

1. A person is treated less favourably than others would be treated or is segregated from others.

2. There is ostensibly equal treatment in that a requirement or condition is applied to all people, but the number of people in a particular racial group who can comply with it is proportionally smaller than the number of people outside that racial group who can comply. (In the act, 'racial group' means a group of persons defined by reference to colour, race, nationality or ethnic or national origins.)
3. Where a person is victimised by being less favourably treated because that person has brought discrimination proceedings, given evidence or information in connection with such proceedings or said that something has been done which would be unlawful under the act.

In relation to job applicants, it is unlawful for employers to discriminate:

1. in recruiting arrangements;
2. in the terms offered with the job; or
3. by not offering the job at all.

In relation to existing employees, it is unlawful for employers to discriminate:

1. in terms of employment;
2. in the way opportunities for promotion, transfer, training or any other benefits are given to employees;
3. by not giving opportunities for promotion, transfer, training or other benefits; or
4. by dismissing an employee or imposing any other penalty on racial grounds.

Race relations employment advisers

The Department of Employment has a number of race relations advisers in the regions of the United Kingdom. These advisers help employers and workers to smooth out difficulties which may arise in a multi-racial workforce. They can be located at Department of Employment regional offices.

There is much controversy about the legislation governing race relations and there is constant argument and testing in the courts of the definitions and terms established by the Race Relations Act. It needs to be said, however, that racial discrimination is wholly abhorrent and should be avoided at all costs by the manager. There is a long tradition in the nursing services of the United Kingdom of recruiting a number of staff from overseas and it is accepted by the majority that the cultural and social mix in the nursing profession is a valuable and useful element.

Complaints of racial discrimination can be particularly traumatic for the individual employee or group of employees concerned and for other members of the workforce. It is imperative that employees from ethnic minorities are treated equitably and fairly.

Sex Discrimination Act 1975

This piece of legislation makes sexual discrimination unlawful in full-time and part-time employment, training and related matters. The act also applies to the conduct of advertising in these areas.

The act explores sexual discrimination against both women and men and against married persons in the field of employment.

Exception where sex is a genuine occupational qualification

Sexual discrimination by an employer in providing access to jobs or training for a job is not unlawful where a person's sex is a genuine occupational qualification for the job under consideration.

Being a man is not generally a genuine occupational qualification for a job. There are a number of provisions where exception is allowed and some examples of this in the nursing service might be where a male nurse or female nurse is required for a particular section of a clinic for sexually transmitted diseases or in a single-sex hospital setting.

The act also amends the Equal Pay Act of 1970; however, since all salary scales in the nursing service are applied equally to both male and female employees, these provisions do not really apply to a nursing situation.

Equal Opportunities Commission

The act established the Equal Opportunities Commission which deals with the duties of working towards the elimination of discrimination, promoting equality of opportunity and keeping under review the working of the Sex Discrimination Act 1975 and the Equal Pay Act 1970.

The commission has the right to promote research in activities of an educational character and in consultation with the Health and Safety Commission will keep under review certain health and safety legislation which requires men and women to be treated differently.

The address of the Equal Opportunities Commission is:

Overseas House,
Quay Street,
Manchester M3 2HN
Telephone: 061-833 9244

The act allows aggrieved employees to take proceedings against an employer through industrial tribunals and the tribunal can:

1. declare the rights of the parties concerned;
2. make a recommendation as to a particular course of action in cases where discrimination is complained of;
3. award compensation on the same basis as the county courts can award damages, but subject to the current limit of unfair dismissal compensation.

The act allows that any compensation awarded may include damages for injured feelings.

The act states that a complaint relating to employment and sex discrimination must be made to a tribunal within three months of the date when the act complained of occurred. However, provision is made for a court or tribunal to consider a complaint, claim or application which is out of time where it is felt just and equitable to do so.

Health and Safety at Work Act 1974

The main provisions of this act are to:

1. maintain or improve standards of health, safety and welfare of persons at work;
2. protect persons other than persons at work against risks to health or safety arising out of or in connection with the activities of persons at work;
3. control and keep the use of explosives or highly flammable or otherwise dangerous substances and generally prevent the unlawful acquisition, possession and use of such substances;
4. control the emission into the atmosphere of noxious or offensive substances from premises of any class prescribed for the purpose of this paragraph; and
5. set up a health and safety commission and executive to be responsible to

the Secretary of State for Employment and other ministers for the administration of this legislation.

Under this act, many of the present regulations relating to health and safety made under previous legislation, for example, the Factories Act of 1961 and Offices, Shops and Railway Premises Act of 1963, are gradually being replaced by new regulations and approved codes of practice enabled under this legislation.

Employers' responsibilities

Under the act, every employer has a duty to ensure the health, safety and welfare at work of all his employees so far as is reasonably practicable. This responsibility should include in particular:

1. the provision and maintenance of plant and systems of work, that are, so far as is reasonably practicable, safe and without risks to health;
2. arrangements for ensuring safety and absence of risks to health in connection with the use, handling, storage and transport of all articles and substances used in the work-place;
3. the provision of instruction, training and supervision as is necessary to ensure, so far as is reasonably practicable, the health and safety at work of his employees;
4. so far as is reasonably practical as regards any place of work under the employer's control, the maintenance of it in a condition that is safe and without risks to health and the provision and maintenance of means of access to and egress from it that are safe and without such risks;
5. the provision and maintenance of a working environment for his employees that is so far as is reasonably practicable, safe, without risks to health and adequate as regards facilities and arrangements for their welfare at work.

These duties are applicable to all senior managers in the National Health Service and employers must prepare a written statement of general policy on health and safety at work related to the needs of their employees and the organisation, and must state arrangements that are in force for carrying out that policy and bring it to the notice of employees.

It is the duty of the employer to consult representatives of the employees with a view to making and maintenance of arrangements which will enable him and his workforce to cooperate effectively in promoting and developing the health and safety at work of employees and in making sure that effective measures are implemented to this end.

The act allows representatives of employees to be appointed by trade unions and these particular safety representatives have the power to request the establishment of safety committees and the employer has no choice in this matter and must accede to such a request.

The act also lays down duties on employers and people who are self-employed to ensure that their activities do not endanger anybody outside their employment and in certain prescribed circumstances to provide information to the public about any potential hazards to health and safety. This section of the act is particularly applicable to hospitals where there are a large number of relatives and other visitors on the premises and it is advisable that provision should be made for this in any local health and safety regulations and agreements.

Employees' responsibilities

Under this act every employee has a duty while at work to take reasonable care for the health and safety of himself and other persons who may be affected by his acts or omissions at work. An employee is also required to cooperate with any duty or requirement imposed on his employer under any of the relevant statutory provisions of the act and to cooperate with him so far as is necessary to enable that duty or requirement to be performed or complied with.

If, for example, a radiotherapy department has a policy for strictly monitoring and controlling the use of radioactive substances, the employee has an absolute duty to comply with the code of practice enforced on the hospital. Another example might be in the handling of cytotoxic drugs and where a health authority has a strict policy for the handling and use of these agents, it is an absolute duty for the employee to comply with policies laid down by management. Failure to comply with such provisions may lead to disciplinary action which could be considered fair in these circumstances.

The Health and Safety Commission

The commission was established in 1974 and consists of a full-time chairman with at least six, and up to nine, part-time members, consisting of representatives drawn from employers' organisations, employees' organisations and other organisations including local authorities. The nine seats on the executive are divided equally between the three groups.

The commission has the power to make whatever arrangements it considers necessary for the purposes of the act. It has to ensure that adequate advice and information on health and safety matters are available and is empowered to undertake research and training as necessary.

It has the duty of preparing new regulations when they are needed and keeps the Secretary of State for Employment informed of its work. The commission also has the duty to carry out directions that are given by the Secretary of State for Employment.

The commission can also arrange for investigations into accidents, incidents or anything else which it considers requires a closer examination. It can also obtain any information needed to carry out its functions. It can also approve and issue codes of practice containing practical guidance made by itself or prepared by other bodies.

The Health and Safety Executive

This body was established in 1975 and consists of a director and two members. It is responsible to the Health and Safety Commission for, in effect, policing the workings of the act. It has a specific duty for making adequate arrangements for the enforcement of the relevant statutory provisions relating to health, safety and welfare in the work-place.

The Health and Safety Executive controls an inspectorate. There are a large number of inspectors throughout the United Kingdom working for the Health and Safety Executive. The health and safety inspector may have a very specific remit, for example, mines and quarries, nuclear installations, etc., or he may have a very generic work-load. Inspectors have very strict powers specified within the act, which are as follows:

1. At any reasonable time or in a situation where the inspector feels it may be dangerous at any time, the inspector has the right to enter any premises which he has reason to believe it is necessary for him to enter and he may examine the whole or any part of those premises and anything within the premises, or to investigate anything which is being done within the premises under inspection.
2. He may take with him a constable if he has reasonable cause to apprehend any serious obstruction in the execution of his duty.
3. He may take with him any other person duly authorised by his enforcing authority and any materials or equipment required for any purpose for which the power of entry is being exercised.

4. He has the right to make such examination or investigation as may, in any circumstances, be necessary.
5. As regards any premises which he has the power to enter, he may direct that those premises or any part of them, or anything within them shall be left undisturbed for so long as is reasonably necessary for the purpose of his examination or investigation.
6. He may take such measurements and photographs and make recordings as he considers fit for the purposes of any examination or investigation.
7. He may take samples of any articles or substances found in any premises which he has the power to enter and he may sample the atmosphere in or around any such premises.
8. In the case of any article or substance which appears to him to have caused or to be likely to cause danger to health or safety, he can have it dismantled or subjected to any process or test, although he is not allowed to damage or destroy it unless it is absolutely necessary.
9. In the case of any such article or substances mentioned in the preceding paragraph, he may take possession of it and detain it for as long as is necessary for all or any of the following purposes, namely:
   (a) to examine it and to do anything which he has the power to do under that paragraph;
   (b) to ensure that it is not tampered with before his examination of it is completed;
   (c) to ensure that it is available for use as evidence in any proceedings for an offence under any of the relevant statutory provisions or any proceedings relating to an improvement or prohibition notice.
10. He has the power to require any person whom he has reasonable cause to believe is able to give any information relevant to examination or investigation to answer such questions as the inspector thinks fit to ask and to sign a declaration of the truth of his answers.
11. He can require the production of, inspect and take copies of any entry in:
    (a) any books or documents which by virtue of any of the relevant statutory provisions are required to be kept, for example, accident books.
    (b) any other books or documents which it is necessary for him to see for the purposes of any examination or investigation under paragraph (4) above.
12. He may ask any person to afford him such facilities and assistance with respect to any matters or things within that person's control or in relation to which that person has responsibilities as are necessary to enable the inspector to exercise any of the powers conferred on him by this section of the act.

13. Any other power which is necessary for the purpose of carrying out his duties.

The inspector can also issue an improvement notice requiring the person believed to be contravening the terms of this act to remedy the contravention within a specified period of time.

If an inspector believes that an activity is so serious that it threatens personal injury, he has the right to issue a prohibition notice. This notice may specify remedial measures to be taken and may either fix a time after which the activity will be prohibited unless such measures are taken, or where the inspector considers that risk of serious injury is imminent he may require the activity to stop immediately until he is satisfied that the cause of risk is remedied.

The inspector has the right to immediately destroy an article or substance if he considers that it is likely to cause imminent personal injury. The act lays down regulations for appeal against improvement or prohibition notices to be made to an industrial tribunal within 21 days of the notice being served.

Inspectors are now assigned to the National Health Service and one can see that it is advisable to take advice from inspectors very seriously indeed. Inspectors will normally be happy to give advice and guidance to managers on any matter related to health and safety in the work-place.

Work-place safety representatives also have a right under the act to approach the inspectorate directly if they are concerned about a particular issue.

The role of the safety representative

The hospital health and safety representative is elected by his colleagues to act as a monitor of health and safety in the work-place on behalf of his colleagues.

Like union stewards, safety representatives are well trained in the basic application of the rules and regulations controlling health and safety in the work-place. All unions in the Health Service have well-established health and safety courses for their representatives and many unions now organise regular refresher courses and updating days as the law relating to health and safety in hospitals grows.

The health and safety representative has a number of important rights under employment law and health and safety legislation. These include:

1. The right to undertake regular health and safety audits of the place of work (this includes ward and departmental areas).

2. The right of access to the health and safety inspectorate for advice or information.
3. The right to expect answers from a management safety officer when the representative brings a hazard in the work-place to the attention of management.
4. The right to adequate information relating to hazards or potential hazards in the work-setting, including access to accident reports.

Health and safety representatives are empowered to make inter-union agreements whereby one union, for example, a non-nursing union, might wish to have an Rcn safety representative acting on behalf of its ancillary members in a ward area. Alternatively, nurses working in small numbers in a scientific or technical department may agree to be represented by a non-nurse. This arrangement was designed to allow for maximum flexibility at local level in response to local needs.

Health and safety at work and nurses

Hospitals are potentially hazardous places to work in. If one considers the number of chemicals and the wide variety of plant and equipment that are to be found on the average hospital site, it is apparent that strict control of health and safety in the work-place is essential.

Hospitals are also full of people from different groups, that is, patients and clients, visitors, and finally, but of equal importance, the staff themselves. The health and safety at work act was brought in with a view to increasing education about the importance of health and safety in the work-setting. It is important to recognise that the penalties contained within the act for transgression of what might be termed good health and safety practice are only there as an ultimate sanction.

The whole philosophy of the act is to increase education and awareness of this important subject. When one looks at accident statistics for staff and patients in hospital settings, it is important that the manager recognises both in financial and human terms the costliness of slack health and safety policies or procedures.

If one begins to think about the potential hazards in a general hospital ward, it becomes clear that nurse managers will increasingly be called upon to define very specifically safe working practices for nursing staff and others in the clinical environment. Lifting and manoeuvring patients, the handling of toxic drugs, the movement and handling of large equipment and machinery related to patient care, the cleanliness of the environment and the safe handling of patients' food are just a few of the examples that are pertinent to any ward area.

The act is relatively new and it will take time for its full impact to be felt within the health service, but it is clear that industry generally and the health service in particular are becoming a good deal more safety-conscious and it is likely that this trend will continue into the future. It is, therefore, essential for nurse managers to be familiar with the main contents of this act and to foster and encourage a healthy attitude towards safety in the work-place.

The safety representative is a key figure at local level and it is sensible for the nurse manager to encourage good relationships with the safety representative. It might also be said that it is prudent to encourage nurses to actively involve themselves in health and safety matters in the work-place.

The local safety representative has a right in law to regularly inspect and carry out safety audits in all areas of the hospital. If there are no nurse health and safety representatives, one could have a situation where non-nurse representatives were attempting to carry out safety audits or inspections at unrealistic times, or at unnecessarily regular intervals, and this could be disruptive to the running of certain clinical areas, for example, intensive care units, renal units, isolation units and medium security units in mental illness/handicap hospitals.

The nurse safety representative will be sensitive to the needs of the patients in certain areas and a good rapport with the safety representative who is also a nurse minimises disruption to the patients and can still allow adequate monitoring of health and safety standards to be maintained.

SUMMARY

Consider the following:

1. Are you as a manager well versed with the basic rules controlling discipline and grievance within your own health authority and your position as a manager under the terms of those agreements?
2. Do you have a system of keeping your knowledge of industrial relations and legislation updated?
3. Does your health authority's personnel department maintain an information centre for nurses in line management, and is this service necessary for nurse managers?
4. Does your health authority have a policy related to disclosure of information to health service trade unions, and have nurse managers in your

authority discussed a policy related to the types of information that might be required by nursing representatives of the trade unions?

5. Does your authority issue written contracts of employment, and are you as a manager familiar with the legal requirements when drafting a written contract of employment?
6. Much new legislation was created during the 1970s and the body of legislation continues to grow. Discuss why this growth in legislation came about and try to think about the advantages and disadvantages in the field of industrial relations and employment law, particularly in the nursing service.

Chapter 5
Case Studies Involving Nurse Managers

RAY ROWDEN

Industrial relations in the nursing service have until recently been relatively tranquil. However, a host of influences have brought about change. In this chapter, I would like to present a number of studies based on my own experience which illustrate how easily the nurse manager can find himself in the midst of the most complicated situations.

Often the most innocent or innocuous circumstances can become major issues which can affect the position of the individual manager and the provision of service in the most dramatic way. *I offer these studies merely as examples and observations to stimulate discussion and thought, and not in any judgemental sense.*

As in so many areas of management, there is no definable right or wrong way to handle a certain matter. It is, however, helpful with the benefit of hindsight to refer to previous experience and to analyse and question our behaviour.

The following studies actually happened, although I have made a number of changes in circumstances in order to protect the identity of the individuals involved. They all occurred within the National Health Service between 1975 and 1980.

THE MISSING WASH BASIN

Mr J was a nursing officer in charge of a small geriatric hospital of 105 beds on the outskirts of a large town. He had worked in the hospital for 17 years from the pre-Salmon days through the 1974 reorganisation of the service, gradually attaining the rank of nursing officer in charge.

He saw himself very much as the matron of the hospital and hung on to certain vestiges of this office. When, for example, the hospital dining room was upgraded, he insisted on keeping his own table where he would be served, whereas all other personnel adapted to a self-service scheme. If he had guests to the hospital, he would lay a superb table in his own spacious office and insist that the catering staff be made available to bring the food from the kitchens up to his office.

He took pride in knowing all of his staff, which consisted of sisters, staff nurses and state-enrolled nurses and a very large proportion of nursing auxiliaries.

His management style was autocratic and the ranking of the nursing hierarchy was strict, with nursing auxiliaries being very definitely at the bottom of the pile. He conducted ward rounds in the old style and expected beds to be in a rigidly straight line. In all, he ran the hospital in a traditional style.

Some of the younger ward sisters seemed to recognise that his style of management was out of step with their experiences elsewhere, but they tolerated him and tried to be loyal to him. The older ward sisters who had grown with him in the hospital accepted his régime and ran their wards according to his style.

Some of the younger, more articulate nursing auxiliaries had joined the union at the hospital and, over a two- or three-year period, became very influential in union affairs. One particular lady became a union shop steward. Through the union machinery, the nursing auxiliaries, who felt a good deal like second-class citizens, began to exercise influence and used local procedures to raise their grievances with the nursing officer. A number of tousles occurred, with the union branch taking on the nursing officer with varying degrees of success.

Mr J reacted to this in a hostile way and felt that the unions had no right to challenge him, least of all nursing auxiliaries. He also resented deeply what he considered to be intrusion from the personnel department, who frequently needed to intervene in the hospital to get Mr J out of various situations.

The nursing auxiliary shop steward broadened her experience by attending TUC and union-sponsored study days and courses and became very adept at using her ancillary colleagues to do her fighting for her. As a result, a constant feeling of mutual dislike and mistrust developed between the nursing auxiliaries and ancillary staff and Mr J.

One evening, Mr J was late leaving work. As he left the main entrance he saw a male domestic worker loading a package wrapped in a hospital polythene bag into the boot of his car. He approached the domestic and enquired as to the contents of the bag. He discovered that the domestic had taken an intact wash basin from a washroom in the hospital that was being refurbished. The domestic had found this basin discarded on a pile of builder's rubble near the site of the work.

Mr J called the hall porter to witness what had happened. The porter was most reluctant to be involved but came when asked. Mr J then insisted that the domestic had to come with him back to his office. The domestic was not at all keen and tried to refuse, but Mr J warned him that he would be in serious trouble if he did not return with him. This was all witnessed by the hall porter.

The domestic eventually went back to the office with Mr J. They spent 20 minutes in the office and the domestic left after the interview in a very distressed state, which he discussed with the hall porter prior to his departure (with the wash basin). The following day an emergency meeting of the union branch was called.

It transpired that the domestic claimed that Mr J had given him a final warning the night before. The domestic claimed that Mr J had told him that if he was ever caught stealing hospital property again, he would lose his job. The union branch was outraged on two counts. First, the domestic supervisor had apparently told the domestic he could have the wash basin since it was no use to the hospital. Second, inspired by the nursing auxiliary shop steward, the branch questioned the whole principle of a nursing officer disciplining a member of the non-nursing staff in this manner. Feelings were running high and it was agreed that the nursing auxiliary shop steward should call the union's regional officer in that afternoon to meet the branch.

The union officer attempted to arrange a meeting with Mr J, who refused to have anything to do with the union. That afternoon the union telephoned the health authority headquarters and told the personnel department that they wanted an urgent meeting convened and that all-out industrial action was a distinct possibility.

The personnel department immediately sent a nurse specialist down to the hospital to interview Mr J. On investigation, Mr J claimed that he had simply wanted to investigate what the male domestic was doing removing property in a hospital bag. He stated that he had simply had stern words with the domestic, but had not disciplined him at all.

Mr J was told that the domestic supervisor had given permission for the basin to be taken. Mr J claimed that the domestic had not told him anything at all about this. The personnel officer then met the union officer and the branch stewards. They were in an irate mood and put forward the following demands. They deprecated the way Mr J had treated their member since it was outside the disciplinary procedure for a manager from the nursing service to discipline a non-nurse. They also stated that Mr J had allowed no opportunity for the domestic to have a friend or representative present to protect his interests. They also resented a false accusation of theft. They advised the nursing personnel officer that the union wanted a written apology from Mr J to the domestic concerned and to the union branch and insisted that Mr J himself be disciplined by higher management for his conduct in the matter. Their final caveat was to advise that strike action would be taken by the branch if these demands were not met.

The personnel nurse asked for time to investigate further and interviewed a number of people involved. The following matters came to light.

The hall porter confirmed that Mr J had been threatening in his attitude towards the domestic at the front of the hospital. The hall porter also claimed that he had heard Mr J shouting loudly at the domestic as he passed Mr J's office door the night before. He was unable to decipher what Mr J had actually said. He reported that the domestic had emerged from the interview in a very distressed state.

The domestic supervisor confirmed that she had told her staff member that she could see no reason why he could not use the basin since the hospital had no possible use for it. However, she denied giving him permission to take it since she had to clear this with the hospital administrator.

The domestic claimed that he had understood that the supervisor had, in fact, given permission. He claimed that he had not told Mr J this because he was so shocked and stunned by the tone of the interview in which he felt he had been warned and disciplined with no recognition of his rights.

The administrator claimed that he had never been approached by the supervisor, but that, had he been, he would have let the staff member have the basin since it was to be disposed of anyway.

There appeared to be a conflict in the disciplinary procedure which had a specific guide to action which may be taken by managers in the nursing and non-nursing groups. The nursing officer was not able to give a nurse anything more than a first written warning, but in the case of extreme misconduct he was able to suspend the staff member pending investigation.

On interview, it transpired that Mr J was totally familiar with the rights of an employee to representation. He maintained that he had not disciplined the domestic. The domestic, however, certainly felt he had been (a) wrongly disciplined, and (b) wrongly accused of theft. The union branch called a full meeting and voted for industrial action if its demands were not met.

Conclusion

The threat of industrial action at the hospital was imminent and the personnel nurse had considered the matter in depth following her investigations. She knew the style of Mr J and had experienced problems with him on previous occasions.

She decided that he had acted wrongly and unwisely in taking the domestic to an office with no witness or representation and advised Mr J accordingly. Her view was that Mr J should have simply suspended the domestic on discovering what appeared to be a misappropriation of hospital property.

She also asked Mr J why he had not removed the wash basin if he had been so concerned about the situation. Mr J could give no explanation to this and simply accused her of backing the unions and allowing the domestic to ride rough-shod over nurse managers.

Meetings were convened to negotiate with the union officer and, following these discussions, the personnel nurse called a meeting with Mr J, the regional officer for the union, the branch secretary and the nursing shop steward.

It had been agreed that Mr J would offer a verbal apology to the individual domestic and to the union, but that nothing would be put into writing.

The personnel nurse refused to allow Mr J to be disciplined but gave a firm assurance to the union that she herself would be supervising all disciplinary matters in the hospital from that day onwards. The union accepted this and action was called off.

In the following months Mr J became extremely bitter about the whole experience and his credibility took a severe blow. The union maximised this and feelings at the hospital remained poor until Mr J eventually retired.

Considerations

1. How would you have managed the situation had you been in Mr J's position?
2. How would you have acted as Mr J's senior officer?
3. How would you have conducted yourself and the enquiry as the personnel nurse specialist?
4. Examine the broader issues in this dispute when a nurse manager may be the most senior person on site after 5 p.m. and at weekends and may have to deal with non-nursing personnel.
5. Examine the position of the union representatives and try to understand why this dispute was important to them.

WHEN TO DISCLOSE AN OFFENCE

Miss T was a student nurse undertaking her SRN training. She was on her second ward after the introductory course and had gained good marks in her theoretical work and received an excellent ward report from her first ward. Prior to entering training she had been employed as a nursing auxiliary in a hospital for the mentally handicapped in a neighbouring authority for a year and had received good references.

One afternoon the senior tutor received an anonymous telephone call from a lady stating that Miss T had been found guilty of shoplifting five years before. The senior tutor tried to gain more information from the caller but the telephone was hung up.

The senior tutor contacted the director of nurse education. They met and discovered that no declaration of any offence had been made on Miss T's original application form. There was, on the form, a clearly worded section asking candidates to declare any convictions.

The director of nurse education contacted the local constabulary who confirmed that Miss T had indeed been found guilty of stealing a large amount of goods from a clothing store and had been placed on probation for one year. She had no previous convictions and had had none since this event.

The director of nurse education and the senior tutor then sent for Miss T and interviewed her, confronting her with the information they had received. Miss T denied the story but the director of nurse education suspended her from duty, pending investigations. In the meantime, Miss T, in a distraught state, contacted her union representative and told the whole story.

The union representative went to the director of nurse education with Miss T and the truth came out and was discussed at length. Miss T explained that the conviction had happened five years previously and at the time of the theft, she was in adolescence and her life at home was extremely unstable. She claimed that she did not declare the offence because it had happened so long ago and that she had avoided further trouble. It also transpired that Miss T had recently been at a party and became involved in a fight. At the party, a girl whom Miss T had known from school days threatened Miss T that she would get even with her. Miss T felt that this girl may have made the anonymous telephone call to the senior tutor.

The director of nurse education challenged Miss T and asked why she had lied when first confronted with the truth and Miss T explained that she was so totally taken aback by the fact that this information had come out and that it was viewed as being of such great importance.

The director of nurse education sought advice from the health authority's headquarters, re-convened the meeting and advised Miss T that she was to be dismissed immediately and paid one month's salary in lieu of notice. The reason given for dismissal was that she had not disclosed the conviction and since nursing was exempt from the provisions of the Rehabilitation of

Offenders Act, her conviction was not spent and should have been accordingly declared on her original application.

Miss T was in great distress and had to tell her family, who knew nothing of the conviction. Her family situation was precarious and she received no support from them at all. On advice from the union representative, Miss T lodged an appeal with the health authority against unfair dismissal.

Conclusion

An appeal hearing before authority members was organised. It was a traumatic affair for all concerned. During the appeal hearing, the director of nurse education and senior tutor were subjected to thorough examination and cross-examination by Miss T's union representative and by the authority members themselves.

It was accepted by the director of nurse education and the senior tutor that Miss T was a good student. Her reports were presented at the hearing and discussed; they supported the view that Miss T was an able student nurse. A ward sister also came to the hearing to testify as a witness on Miss T's behalf.

The union unearthed details of previous cases involving nurses in the authority's employment who had been found guilty of theft, but who had not been sacked. There were, however, no precedents to be found involving the non-declaration of an offence prior to employment.

After a long and arduous hearing, the authority panel upheld the decision of the director of nurse education to dismiss Miss T and advised her accordingly. Miss T left nursing and eventually found alternative employment. She had no recourse to an industrial tribunal because her continuous service was not sufficient to allow her this right.

Considerations

1. How would you as a manager react to anonymous information of this nature?
2. Are you familiar with the provisions of the Rehabilitation of Offenders Act and its effects on nursing?
3. How would you have handled this case if you were in the position of the director of nurse education?
4. Discuss the implications and possible consequences for the director of nurse education and the health authority had they decided not to dismiss Miss T and taken less severe disciplinary action.

A MANAGER OVERRULED

Mrs S was a divisional nursing officer in a large hospital for the mentally handicapped. She was an experienced manager and had qualifications and experience in many areas of nursing, but had chosen mental handicap as her first love. She had been appointed divisional nursing officer in 1975 and had been happy in her position.

Her senior nursing officer reported to her that a group of nursing auxiliaries had made serious allegations against a senior ward sister involving her conduct on the ward on her birthday. The nursing auxiliaries stated that the ward sister had been under the influence of alcohol and had behaved in an outrageous manner, throwing food around, making suggestive sexual advances towards a male nurse, dipping a junior nurse into the ward bath and eventually collapsing in the staff room to sleep off the effects of her celebration, vomiting in a sink *en route* and leaving the ward in the care of junior untrained nurses.

Mrs S was shocked to hear of these revelations and immediately sent for the ward sister for interview. There had been a considerable time lapse between the ward sister's birthday and the actual reporting of these incidents from the auxiliary staff.

At interview, the ward sister seemed utterly shocked at the allegations. Mrs S decided to suspend the ward sister on full pay and conduct a full investigation. Statements were taken from all parties and a hearing was established where the ward sister was represented by her union. Mrs S had the support of her senior nursing officer and a personnel officer at this hearing. At interview and examination of the witnesses, the following matters came to light.

There was some conflict in evidence as to the amount of alcohol the ward sister had actually consumed on the day in question. Some witnesses overstated the ward sister's behaviour and attributed it to her being drunk, others suggested that it was simply horseplay that had gone a little too far. There was only one witness to the ward sister supposedly vomiting in the sink and falling asleep; no other witnesses saw the sister asleep in the staff room. Mrs S in discussion with the senior nursing officer, personnel officer and union representative, weighed up the case. It appeared that there was a reasonable amount of collective animosity between the ward sister and certain witnesses, and that there was a risk that some of the witnesses could have collaborated in a conspiratorial way against the ward sister.

Mrs S was disturbed by the incongruity of the stated severity of the ward sister's behaviour and the time it actually took for the nursing auxiliaries to report the matter. Mrs S had no doubt that there was some substance to the allegations and that even if the ward sister's behaviour was only horseplay going too far, she had still behaved very badly and was responsible for the example she set to her junior staff.

The ward sister concerned was not the most dynamic person in the hospital but, on the other hand, she had a stable record with no serious problems. Mrs S decided that the ward sister's conduct was serious enough to warrant a final written warning under the terms of the disciplinary procedure, and also decided to move the ward sister to another clinical area where she could have a period of much closer supervision from a nursing officer. This was discussed with the senior nursing officer and personnel officer and their decisions were then presented to the ward sister and her union representative who accepted that the decision was fair, given the total circumstances.

On the following day, Mrs S was summoned to the office of the chief nursing officer of the authority and told that the matter was being taken out of her hands. Mrs S was astonished since the authority had a clear written procedure which detailed her sphere of action in disciplinary matters. As far as she was concerned, she had acted in accordance with the policy and had taken the right managerial decision. She was advised that the ward sister concerned would be dismissed from employment and reported to a statutory body. The chief nurse also warned that he was considering taking action against Mrs S herself for her handling of the affair. Mrs S was thrown into a dilemma since she felt that her handling of the matter had been appropriate and fair. The ward sister was duly dismissed and lodged an appeal to the health authority.

At appeal, Mrs S had to be totally honest and the union representative for the ward sister made it known to the authority panel of members that there was a severe split between senior managers over this matter.

The ward sister's appeal was upheld and she was reinstated on full pay pending investigation by the statutory body. Mrs S felt in a very uncomfortable position, knowing that the authority had, in effect, supported her decision against that of the chief nurse.

Some months passed while the ward sister awaited a date for a hearing at the statutory body. At that hearing, it was decided to take action against the ward sister and her name was removed from the register. At the hearing, however, the authority was heavily criticised, particularly for the lack of a clear policy on the position of nurses using alcohol in a work-setting.

On losing her qualifications, the ward sister was no longer able to fulfil her contract of employment and her contract was terminated by the authority. The statutory body was sympathetic to the ward sister's position, but felt that it was in her own best interests to remove her from clinical practice for a period of time. After the event, the chief nurse took steps against Mrs S which led to much trauma and acrimony.

Considerations

1. Is there a need for a clear policy on the subject of alcohol consumption while on duty?
2. Does your own authority have such a policy for nursing staff, and if so, does it provide sufficient clarity for employees and managers?
3. How would you have reacted as a manager to your instructions being overruled by a more senior officer?
4. Is there adequate provision for this type of situation in procedure documents?
5. Who should have the right to decide when a nurse is to be reported to a statutory body and should this decision be vested in the hands of the chief nurse or the authority itself with nursing advice?

WHAT CONSTITUTES REASONABLE TIME OFF FOR UNION ACTIVITIES?

Mr X was a health visitor and an active union steward. He served as district convener for his local stewards and also served on a regional authority committee and a national committee of his own union. During a pay campaign, he had to attend many meetings, both within the authority and within his own union. This detracted from his work. At routine times he usually took the equivalent of approximately one working day each month in order to meet his various union commitments. Much of his union activity was done in his own time by re-scheduling his workload. This he was able to do as a health visitor.

As the pay campaign gathered momentum, his union workload increased dramatically. Some non-nurse unionists were planning industrial action and he was having to attend many meetings to coordinate the position of his nurse members during the dispute. This necessitated him taking up to one day a week attending various meetings at local and regional level.

Mr X had always had an informal arrangement with local management and had given notice to his immediate line manager when he needed to absent himself from work. During the dispute he had to attend emergency meetings locally at very short notice. His nursing officer had to ask some colleagues to cover certain commitments on his case load with very little warning.

His colleagues had not complained about this, but his nursing officer expressed concern to more senior managers. As the dispute intensified, Mr X was requested to attend an urgent meeting at his union headquarters in London. He gave his nursing officer ten days' advance warning that he wished to attend this meeting at national level. His nursing officer explained that she would have to seek permission for him to attend the meeting, saying that one day a week was more than enough time and that since this meeting was at a national level and not related to local matters, it was not reasonable for him to be allowed time off to attend.

Mr X maintained that he had given management ten days' notice of his wish to attend the meeting and claimed that this was perfectly reasonable. He also stated that although the meeting was at a national level, the conduct of the dispute and his input through his union did bear relevance to the situation in his own authority.

Mr X sought advice from his union office, who advised him of his right to reasonable time off for trade union duties under conditions of employment legislation and under the terms of his own authority's policy statement, which was agreed by the local joint consultative committee which consisted of management and trade union representatives. This agreement only said that requests for reasonable amounts of time off for union officials would not be unreasonably refused. The trade union officer contacted the health authority headquarters and the chairman of the authority's labour relations panel, and stated that it would be taking the matter to industrial tribunal and that Mr X would also invoke the grievance procedure which had also been negotiated by the consultative committee. This action was put into effect and Mr X advised his nursing officer that since a formal grievance had been lodged, the status quo position should be maintained and that he would be taking time off to attend the meeting.

The nursing officer contacted the divisional nursing officer for the community services who discussed the matter with the chief nurse of the authority. The chief nurse sought advice on the matter from the nurse personnel officer who advised that Mr X could face disciplinary action if he attended without permission. The divisional nursing officer convened a meeting with Mr X in the presence of the nursing officer and another steward representing Mr X. At the interview, the divisional nursing officer quoted an industrial tribunal judgement relating to a nurse who was refused time off to attend a meeting at national level. She claimed that the tribunal had ruled that it was reasonable for an authority to refuse permission for an employee to attend a meeting at a national level.

Mr X stated that his individual case might well be different in substance from the case quoted and that the status quo provision should allow him to attend the meeting in the knowledge that a judgement on his grievance and judgement from an industrial tribunal would give a decision one way or the other. He also offered to use a day's annual leave should the grievance hearing and tribunal judgement go against him.

The divisional nursing officer stated that this was not the point and that it was a matter of principle that he could not absent himself from work without her permission. She advised him that if he were to do so, he could face severe disciplinary action. Mr X asked her if he was being given an informal warning and she stated that this was not the case and that she just wished to discuss the matter with him. He stated that he felt that he had been threatened and advised the divisional nursing officer that he would be contacting his union's full-time officer. The meeting ended on a very acrimonious note with the divisional nursing officer and Mr X both losing their tempers and exchanging harsh words. The situation was going from bad to worse and the union officer asked the authority's administrator to convene a hearing to hear Mr X's grievance immediately.

The administrator contacted the chairman of the authority's labour relations panel, and, after discussion, it was agreed that a panel of authority members would be convened to consider the case on the following day.

Conclusion

At the hearing, Mr X was represented by his union officer. The nursing officer gave evidence which showed the dramatic increase in Mr X's time off for union duties during the period of the dispute. She also quoted a number of occasions where she had had to provide cover for Mr X's clients at very short notice indeed.

The nursing officer confirmed that she and Mr X had always had an informal arrangement and that there had never been any problems prior to this occasion. The divisional nursing officer stated at the hearing that provision of service to clients was the first duty of the authority and that she felt it was not vital for Mr X to attend the meeting in London since he had received enough time off to cover his duties at local and regional level.

The trade union officer put his case and claimed that Mr X had been perfectly reasonable in giving his managers ten days' notice of a meeting at national level. He claimed that this meeting was crucial to the management of the pay dispute and that Mr X's professional knowledge was essential in the coordination of the union's nursing membership if patients were not to suffer dangerously during planned industrial action. He stated that this had direct relevance to the health authority. Mr X called two fellow health visitors who testified that they had never complained to management about having to cover his case load, and that they understood his position as a union representative.

The trade union officer called the shop steward who had accompanied Mr X to the meeting with the divisional nursing officer and the nursing officer and who had taken notes at that meeting. The trade union officer tried to show that the divisional nursing officer had, in effect, threatened Mr X with disciplinary action and that this constituted an informal warning. The trade union officer quoted employment law which states that no disciplinary action can be taken against a union official related to his union activities unless a senior official of the union is notified.

The authority's panel adjourned to consider the case and returned the following decision. They decided that management had been unreasonable in refusing to allow time off since Mr X had given ten days' notice; they were also cognisant of the fact that the authority lacked a detailed policy on this matter and felt it fair to give Mr X the benefit of the doubt on this occasion, given a lack of clear policy.

They also stated that they had been impressed by Mr X's willingness to take the day off as annual leave. They, therefore, overruled the manager's decision and gave Mr X permission to attend the meeting.

They rejected the claim that Mr X had been disciplined and also stated that since this matter had not been notified as part of his original grievance, they could not and would not consider it further.

The hearing was closed and the panel privately conveyed criticism to the divisional nursing officer over her handling of the interview with Mr X and his fellow shop steward. The divisional nursing officer felt distressed by the whole experience and felt that she had been personally betrayed by her employing authority. The chief nursing officer for the authority shared her view and conveyed this to the chairman of the panel. The matter went no further. In the following months, the labour relations panel of the authority asked the joint consultative committee to negotiate a more specific agreement related to time off for union activities which could be considered by the full authority.

Considerations

1. Are you, as a manager, familiar with the legislation and Whitley Council agreements relating to time off for trade union activities?

2. Does your own authority have a policy related to this subject? Is this policy general and vague or quite specific?
3. Consider the advantages and disadvantages of a specific and detailed agreement on this subject. Are specific and detailed policies feasible, practical or necessary in the nursing service?
4. How would you have handled this situation as the divisional nursing officer?
5. How would you have handled the situation as the chairman of the panel hearing the case?
6. What do you consider to be a reasonable amount of time off for a senior union steward who is a nurse? Ask colleagues the same question and compare your views.

HOW MUCH EVIDENCE DOES A MANAGER NEED TO TAKE ACTION?

Sister V was an experienced psychiatric nurse who had worked in a number of areas of her hospital. She had 20 years of nursing experience behind her. The nursing managers considered her to be traditional in her approach to her work but totally reliable.

She always ran her ward well in their eyes and would often go and help out on other wards when there was a lack of qualified staff. Over a two-year period, the divisional nursing officer had heard occasional mutterings via the School of Nursing that students and pupils did not like working with her. It appeared that her régime was considered to be institutionalised and uncaring, fostering only a custodial approach to care.

A male student nurse approached his personal tutor with a catalogue of complaints against this particular sister. He claimed that she was bullying and overbearing to certain patients, who were considered by her to be a nuisance. He also claimed that Sister V used frequent slaps to correct the behaviour of long-stay patients, and that she frequently overmedicated patients with major tranquillisers and locked them in side wards for long periods of time, often depriving them of food or facilities for using the toilet.

The student was greatly disturbed by what he claimed he had seen. The tutor approached the divisional nursing officer, who decided to interview the student with his union representative. The divisional nursing officer questioned the student very closely and eventually suggested that the student's perception of events was influenced by his lack of experience and that he had misjudged Sister V.

The student refused to accept this interpretation completely. The divisional nursing officer then asked the student nurse if he wished to make a formal complaint. The student stated that he did wish to do so, and he was advised by the divisional nursing officer to put his complaint into writing.

On the following day, the divisional nursing officer received a written statement from the student which itemised his complaints. The student gave examples of Sister V's misconduct. The letter also named certain patients and other members of the ward staff who had supposedly witnessed Sister V's maltreatment. The divisional nursing officer discussed the matter with the administrator, and it was decided that the statement should be referred to the police, since some of the allegations involved assault against patients.

Sister V was seen by the divisional nursing officer and suspended from duty pending the outcome of enquiries by the police. Word spread through the hospital like wildfire and rumours circulated.

Sister V was well established in the hospital and served on the staff social club committee, organising many social events. A strong sense of loyalty developed around her and she received many visits, letters and telephone calls, all of a sympathetic nature. The divisional nursing officer also received many similar overtures from many members of the staff. Middle managers all supported Sister V totally and felt sure that the student's lack of experience lay at the root of the complaints.

The police took the student nurse to the station and obtained a full and detailed statement from him. They came into the hospital on numerous occasions and carried out a large number of interviews with ward staff. Sister V was also interviewed at length, as were a number of long-stay patients who were considered fit for interview by the consultant psychiatrist. The police also had access to patients' case records and studied the records of the patients who had been mentioned by the student nurse. The whole process was lengthy and extremely traumatic for all concerned.

Feeling in the hospital was running high and many staff expressed mistrust and resentment towards the student concerned, although this was never directly aimed at the student.

When the police interviewed staff on the ward, no-one was able or willing to give evidence to support the student nurse's claims. The patients' records showed no signs of irregularity and the hospital pharmacy records could ot show any vast discrepancies or inconsistencies. The student had claimed that Sister V frequently doubled the doses of major tranquillisers for some patients and often gave large injections as punishments to certain patients.

Throughout the next five weeks, the student went through a great deal of pressure and received little or no support from anyone apart from his personal tutor. He felt ostracised but insisted that he had told the truth and that he trusted the evidence of his own eyes. A nursing officer approached him on two occasions and asked him to withdraw his allegations.

Following police enquiries, the divisional nursing officer was advised that proceedings against Sister V would not be taken due to the lack of evidence. Sister V was then allowed to return to work on the same ward with no further action.

The divisional nursing officer saw her before her return and made it plain that he was delighted with the outcome of the police enquiries. Sister V's colleagues around the hospital were equally delighted and she returned to the bosom of the hospital. No further managerial action was considered necessary or taken. The student nurse resigned shortly afterwards. The hospital was at ease once more and returned to its own normality.

For the next two years, Sister V remained in the same ward. She was perceived in the same manner by her superiors and all seemed well. Her ward was still known to be disliked by students, but nothing specific was ever mentioned or reported.

At this time, a new young nursing auxiliary was sent to Sister V's ward. After three months the nursing auxiliary decided to discuss Sister V's attitude and behaviour with a student nurse who was on the ward. The auxiliary expressed her concern at events she had witnessed and felt able to trust the student. They met off duty and discussed their misgivings at length and decided to take some action since they had both seen certain types of misconduct and abuse, although it transpired that they were never present together to witness this. The student approached the tutor who had been involved in the previous incident with Sister V.

The tutor interviewed the nursing auxiliary and student nurse together and was horrified at what they had to tell him. Their catalogue of complaints was very similar in substance to those outlined two years previously by the lone student nurse who had given up his training after Sister V's return to work.

The tutor advised the student and auxiliary of the seriousness of their allegations and warned them of what might ensue if they put in a formal complaint. They went away and considered their position and decided to see the divisional nursing officer.

The divisional nursing officer interviewed them separately and, again, suggested that they were young and inexperienced and that they might be simply misjudging what they had seen because of this. He expressed sympathy and understanding of their position, but felt that this was probably what had happened. Their complaints were almost identical in content to those of the original student nurse. The student and the auxiliary persisted with their claims and put them into writing.

The divisional nursing officer again discussed the matter with the hospital administrator, but it was decided that, on this occasion, no police involvement was needed until an internal enquiry had examined the matter in depth. Sister V was advised of the allegations and was allowed to remain on duty.

During the next fortnight, the divisional nursing officer and administrator interviewed a large number of staff. None of their statements supported the evidence of the auxiliary and the student. Following a period of investigation, the divisional nursing officer and administrator established a hearing involving themselves and one member of the consultant medical staff.

It was agreed that all parties would be represented and the matters raised by the junior staff could be examined in depth. The hearing lasted for two days and involved union representatives acting for Sister V and for the student and auxiliary.

During the hearing, Sister V's representative made great play of the fact that no other staff had witnessed the alleged misconduct. He also stressed that neither of the two witnesses had been on duty together to see anything, and during cross-examination of the student nurse and auxiliary it became clear that they were somewhat vague about the dates and times of the alleged incidents.

The divisional nursing officer and administrator saw some of the patients in the ward, who had no complaints to make.

After the enquiry, it was decided that there was no corroborative evidence to support the claims of the two junior staff members and that their complaints were found to be not proven.

The members of the enquiry panel told the student and auxiliary that they understood their position as younger, less-experienced members of staff and that they wanted to reassure them that they were correct in reporting their disquiet at what they had misunderstood. Sister V had no action taken against her, but the divisional nursing officer saw her privately and warned her to watch her conduct in the presence of younger members of the staff. She was also moved to another ward in the hospital. A report of the enquiry and the events leading up to it was sent to the authority. In that report, no mention was made of any previous complaint against Sister V. This report was accepted.

During the period of complaints and investigations, Sister V received exactly the same loyalty from her colleagues that she had received two years previously. Again, rumour became rife and tension within the hospital ran high.

After the internal enquiry, there was some dissatisfaction that Sister V had to be moved from her own ward. Things soon, however, returned to normal in the hospital. The nursing auxiliary resigned shortly afterwards and found another job but the student nurse continued training.

Conclusion

Shortly after these events, the local community health council was approached by the nursing auxiliary who had resigned. The nursing auxiliary gave information relating to the behaviour of the sister at the hospital and also complained about many other aspects of the running of the long-stay wards within the hospital.

The auxiliary advised the community health council that there was a core of younger staff members who could support her evidence, but they were all afraid to come forward. The community health council had little or no cooperation from the hospital during visits and had expressed concern to the district management team about the standards of care at the hospital for a considerable period of time.

The district management team had always supported the hospital managers. On receipt of a signed statement from the auxiliary, and following further interviews with other staff members, the community health council compiled a dossier and sent it to the regional health authority and the Secretary of State for Health.

The issue leaked to the press and the hospital became the focus of much public attention. The situation became more heated and the regional health authority established a full committee of enquiry which was to report publicly. Over the next year, the hospital was subjected to a full-scale enquiry, involving the taking of hundreds of statements and the examination of many witnesses. The enquiry criticised the divisional nursing officer for his handling of the complaints against Sister V, and suggested that it was wrong of him to have let matters rest simply because the police investigations had revealed no evidence of criminal conduct.

The enquiry panel made it plain that they were highly critical of the whole episode. The enquiry uncovered many other aspects of poor standards within the hospital and the whole experience was traumatic for the hospital staff, and rather sad for the divisional nursing officer, who had to end a long career on a very sour note indeed.

Considerations

1. How would you have approached the original student's complaints as: (a) the nurse tutor, or (b) the divisional nursing officer?
2. Examine the legal issues and the professional issues involved in the case. Is there a difference between the two?
3. Is it vital for two witnesses to be available in cases of alleged misconduct before a manager can take action?
4. Examine the concept of institutional loyalty towards long-standing members of staff. Could this influence your judgement as a manager in an inappropriate way?
5. Examine the reasons as to why no other witnesses came forward to support the complaints of the student in the case.
6. Do you think management could have prevented the necessity for a full-scale enquiry?
7. Do external enquiry teams have any value to a hospital and what should nursing management's attitude be towards such enquiries?

Chapter 6
Managing Manpower

PETER BREARLEY

The manner in which individuals and organisations approach the management of their personnel varies considerably. This difference of approach arises from their interpretation of what constitutes 'personnel', plus the influence which its historical development has had upon them. To many the term 'personnel management' includes all those aspects of managerial function which have a direct bearing on the management of human resources within the organisation. Some managers and staff representatives will not wholly agree with a description of that nature and would see the management of human resources as a total concept, within which personnel management is only one aspect alongside training, industrial relations and some elements of industrial psychology. The split is immaterial; what is important is to indicate the importance of the manager's activity in utilising the human resources which he controls.

The way in which the maximum utilisation of those human resources is achieved is as important as the actual achievement and will reflect, to some extent, the priorities which a particular organisation holds. It is unlikely that any manager will be able to realise the maximum potential of the resources under his direction if he pursues a style of personnel management relating only to the provision of an industrial relations service on a 'fire-fighting' basis. A planned, forward-looking approach to the management of expensive human resources can only be successfully achieved if the policies of the organisation on all the major aspects of personnel are clear. Such policies need to be clear not only to line managers and personnel professionals; they also need to be clear to the staff being managed. It is for this reason that clear policy statements in the field of personnel are so important, particularly in a large organisation like the National Health Service where the managed groups on average tend to be larger than in industry or commerce, with all the attendant possibilities of misinterpretation and misunderstandings, leading to grievance and even industrial dispute.

Any policies which the manager seeks to bring into operation affecting staff groups should endeavour to accomplish at least three things: first, they should meet all legal requirements which apply to the employment of staff and the manner in which they work. Secondly, they should reflect the manner in which the employing authority wishes the service to develop, including the way in which the authority requires its staff to be managed. Thirdly, they should form a practical and sensible guide to employment practices, allowing the manager and the staff involved to carry out the commitments of the employing authority in the delivery of health care.

Policies, however well written and detailed they may be in meeting legal requirements, will, if they fail to allow the organisation to carry out its task in the delivery of care in the most effective way, prove problematic sooner or later and are to be avoided.

Table 2 Some areas of personnel management requiring policy statements.

1. Training
2. Advertising
3. Retirement
4. Equal opportunities
5. Health and safety at work
6. Discipline *v.* dismissal
7. Grievances
8. Facilities for trade union activities
9. Absence due to injury and ill health

Examples of some of the areas requiring policy statements are shown in Table 2. Establishing such policies will allow the managers to concentrate on a planned progressive improvement of services allied to an improved efficiency in the management of human resources without disadvantaging individuals or groups of staff within their organisation.

Once an organisation or an individual manager, by the allocation of inadequate resources, lack of interest or poor practice, allows the personnel aspect of management to move into the arena of 'fire-fighting' activities – it will become increasingly difficult and costly for the organisation to recapture lost ground. For any nurse manager moving to a new employer or department in the NHS, time spent on the development of their personnel practices early on in their appointment will pay large dividends at a later date. The manager who fails to do this will regret it for years to come.

Before a manager decides on an area of personnel activity, it is best to obtain a clear indication from seniors as to the short- and long-term priorities of the service they are to manage. This may seem an obvious step to advocate but in the days of very limited resources only clearly understood priorities can warrant the expenditure of time and effort. An example of how the priorities might affect personnel activities lies in considering some opposites. In a newly commissioned hospital, a considerable amount of time and effort will need to be put into the area of recruitment. This is different from a hospital which is undergoing a changing role: here perhaps the majority of the personnel manager's time will be involved in the management of change, including the retraining of staff.

A third and different proposition is where a manager is required to reduce an area of existing service, possibly by the closure of facilities. In this case, a considerable amount of personnel effort will need to go into such areas as the reallocation of staff, preparation of redundancy agreements and management of working arrangements during the run-down period. None of these areas of emphasis can possibly be efficiently managed without an early understanding of the service's priorities.

The manager's decision on how to proceed in developing the personnel function, whether as a line manager or the user of a personnel service, will be moulded by the manner in which the function has developed, the locality, the manager's own experience of personnel work and equally important the limitations imposed on personnel development by resource availability. The history of the personnel function within the NHS is a chequered one, its major development having taken place since the 1974 reorganisation. For nursing, this has tended to result in the appointment of nurses with authority-wide responsibility in personnel work, reflecting the 1974 reorganisation recommendation for the appointment of Area Nurses (Personnel).

The background of the individuals appointed differed greatly. In the early days only a small number were personnel professionals. Their knowledge varied from a recognised course of training and qualification, to entry directly from service posts, without personnel training and sometimes without any experience of personnel management. It has only been by the foresight of some authorities and the efforts of many that the personnel management skills of nurses developed significantly prior to the restructuring of 1982.

The overall personnel function, spearheaded by Area and District personnel officers, has also developed in the main since 1974, although there were some 'establishment' and particularly medical 'establishment' officers prior to 1974. Difficult industrial relations in the NHS and increasing involvement in the introduction of incentive systems for ancillary workers, combined with major changes in legislation during the 1970s, provided the incentive to develop personnel management within Health Authorities. Unfortunately, there is still a considerable difference in the level of facilities and expertise offered by personnel departments to individual managers.

Where an individual nurse manager does not have a substantial amount of experience in the management of staff, for example, he/she may be moving into line management from predominantly clinical posts or moving into a post where the duties and working environment are drastically different, then they would be well advised not only to seek support from their local personnel department but also to undertake an assessment of their needs with a view to securing an adequate personnel service. To specify one's requirements in this way will lead to one of two things happening: either one will receive adequate support particularly during the early period of the appointment or one will be able to identify the shortfall. It is helpful to establish the requirement of the manager; it is not always easy to persuade people to change the allocation of resources once the pattern is set.

The most pressing limitation on provision of personnel services is not industrial legislation or lack of interest, but the shortage of resources for the development of services to meet growing patient needs and expectations.

THE STRUCTURE OF PERSONNEL SERVICES

For most nurse managers, the structure of the service will have been dictated before they arrive on the scene and in many instances will not change significantly in the near future. However, it is wrong to assume that there are not different approaches available in terms of structuring a personnel service and these need to be considered against resource limitations. The limitations in cash terms are important although the availability of personnel skills will also be a major consideration, as to a lesser extent will physical accommodation for those providing the service.

Many individuals will wish to consider their structure in terms of centralised personnel departments supporting managers in the field. This approach allows what are often rare skills and resources to be used effectively by retaining them together and making them available throughout the authority. It reduces duplication of work and equipment and goes some way towards ensuring a single approach to priorities and policies throughout the service. However, it is not popular with all nurse managers because they feel that a centralised service can in some instances be distant and slow to react to their individual managerial requirements. It is also sometimes criticised on the basis that it develops an 'us and them' situation between the line manager and personnel function. Alternatively, unit level personnel staff alongside the line managers helps to identify personnel specialists within the managed unit and solidifies the management approach.

Some Authorities have considered, and introduced, a mixture of unit personnel services with central support. This normally works on the basis of out-posting to each major unit within the Authority a very small number of personnel staff – often only one individual who is not normally of a high grade. These individuals give day-to-day support to line managers in prescribed areas of work while themselves receiving specialist support from a small central core facility. A number of line managers like this option because it gives them on-the-spot personnel assistance, it is easier to identify with and ensures a quicker response to the needs of the managed unit.

The third option is to provide a unit-based personnel staff without a central support facility. In order to do this adequately and maintain effective communication with the units a considerable amount of inter-unit organisation is necessary. It is also perhaps the most costly way of providing a personnel service. Where this happens there is, of course, always the risk that the post at unit level will not be adequately graded to attract people of sufficient calibre. A reduced area of experience may result, which will leave each unit to find its own way of resolving personnel problems, with the possibility of reinventing the wheel several times a year.

Problems may also arise particularly in areas such as non-professional training, where the smaller units will not have available the necessary resources or indeed the necessary demand to run some courses economically. Any of the problems which have been noted above can result in a deterioration of personnel service throughout the Health Authority.

It would be wrong not to consider the line managers as personnel managers; indeed, all managers who control groups of staff are in themselves personnel managers. The main difference between these and personnel staff working in personnel departments is the degree of training, knowledge and experience of various aspects of personnel. However, there is no reason why an individual manager should not be able to provide his own complete personnel service providing he is adequately trained and has an adequate amount of time available to do this. Above all he must see human resource management as being the major aspect of his work. Given the intricacies of present employment law, the law on health and safety at work, the cost of providing training for small groups of staff and the need to provide 'whole authority' policies as part of maintaining a corporate identity, it is unlikely that line managers without personnel department support will be efficient and economic in the management of staff.

In the case of large units and particularly in relation to nursing services, the concept of unit personnel nurses answerable on a day-to-day basis to the line manager while relating on personnel issues to a central personnel department is well worth pursuing as it tends to offer the line manager the best of both worlds.

SOME MAJOR ASPECTS OF PERSONNEL WORK

The aspects of personnel work which are seen within a particular organisation as being the most time-consuming will change considerably over a given period as will their relative importance. This is only right and will normally be a reflection of the priorities within the authority and of the changing employment environment, including the changes in legislation. The success of a personnel manager might indeed be judged in terms of the ability to respond to the changing environment. Failure to be able to respond or a lack of understanding of the management of change will bring with it many problems. However, it is perhaps reasonable to suggest that some of the following areas do constitute the main aspects of personnel work within the NHS or any other large organisation. What will change considerably is the emphasis which is placed on each activity at different times.

Advertising and recruitment

In many cases nurse managers see the first step in obtaining staff as being the placement of an advertisement. It is here that many of the problems in recruitment first occur. The first step should be taken long before placing an advertisement and should deal with the question of analysing the needs of the organisation. I would suggest that some simple questions need to be asked before one even starts to describe the type of individual one hopes to recruit:

1. Does the job that the previous job holder was doing actually need to be done at all?
2. If it does need to be done, can it be done by someone else or by a group of other people already in the authority's employ?
3. Is it desirable to do the work in a different way to the way in which it is done now?
4. If it can be done by others, would this make it more expensive or cheaper?

Only if, as a result of asking these questions, one is assured that the job will be best carried out by an individual not currently in the organisation's employment should there be any question of moving on to the next stage in the recruitment process, which is to draw up a job description.

It is not adequate to reissue standard job descriptions for posts. Every job description should reflect the specific job that is to be done. It will be a record of the facts relating to the post to be filled and may be conveniently divided into such sections as professional responsibilities, personnel responsibilities and managerial responsibilities. It is often a good idea to include with the job description a note of what the employer sees as the key task; this might be reasonably done on a sheet which also outlines the reporting arrangements. Sample job descriptions are available from a number of well-established personnel management books, as is detailed advice on the writing of job descriptions.

Once the job description has been completed, the manager can attempt to identify from that job description a picture of the type of individual that will be required to fulfil the needs of the job description. This is the opportunity to identify the qualifications which the applicant is required to hold, to note the necessary experience required to carry out the duties of the post in question and to consider such items as whether the individual should live on the premises or close to his work base, which can be important if on-call and rota duties apply. It is also an opportunity to specify such things as further training requirements where it is believed that the market will not yield an individual with all the experience/qualifications that would be expected of the 'perfect applicant'.

The part of the exercise sometimes known as drawing up the 'man specification' is very important; not only does it give the manager the chance to clarify in his own mind the type of individual being sought, it also provides a blueprint against which the interviewing checklist can be set. If a picture is not drawn up in this way, there is no way in which one can realistically weight the attributes which are being sought in an applicant. The result of this is that very unspecific ideas are held by the interviewing panel, such as 'must be SRN, medical ward experience desirable' – there must be many thousands of qualified nurses who could fit that 'man specification', but whether any of them really meets the requirement of the post which is to be filled is another matter.

Once the job description and 'man specification' have been written we can then turn to the question of advertising and recruitment. Many people are of the opinion that they can quite ably draw up advertisements which will yield the type of applicants they hope to attract, but in experience this is often far from the truth. Therefore, one of the first considerations needs to be whether or not the assistance of an advertising agency should be employed or some other form of specialist advice sought.

Many Personnel Departments will have on their staff people with experience of advertising who will be quite capable of drawing up advertisements which are likely to attract an adequate number of relatively qualified and experienced applicants. However, it must be accepted that there are areas in nursing, as in other professional groups, where, however good or expensive the advertising (the two do not necessarily go together), the yield in terms of enquiries will be limited. These groups are often referred to as 'shortage specialties' and here alternatives must be sought in filling vacancies. Alternatives may include casting a wider recruitment net, retraining of individuals within the organisation, or possibly setting up long-term training programmes on the basis of developing one's own nurses for that specialty. The latter course is quite costly but in some instances is the only course of meaningful action that is open to the nurse manager.

Let us turn our attention then to the advertisement itself. The essential core information for any advertisement is that which allows the reader to know what the job is, whom they will be working for, that is, who is the employer, what type of person is being looked for and, in the case of the nurse, what are any required or preferred qualifications. It should allow potential applicants to understand fairly clearly what the remuneration/benefits of the post are, and where it is located. One common source of disappointment for applicants occurs when they apply to a central department situated, for instance, in a District General Hospital, which they find it easy to travel to, only to discover at interview that the post exists in a peripheral unit. The advertisement should also include an indication of the action individuals must take if they wish to apply for the post.

To this core information can be added the principle of providing an advertisement that is attractive. However, this does not mean that the best results will always be obtained through providing high-quality artwork or massive headlines. It is usually the combination of good presentation and meaningful information which attracts the would-be employee.

One part of an advertisement that is always worth considering, particularly in a new or developing service, is whether there is any aspect of the job which is different to traditional posts using the same title. This could be particularly meaningful in the employment of nurse therapists, community nurses, or nurses who are taking on a new role associated with a changing pattern of care. The result of including an indication of this in the advertisement may well be to encourage more forward-looking professionals to apply in the hope that this is a job which will give them not only a new experience, but increased job satisfaction.

Managers should endeavour to keep a record of the response to advertisements previously placed, a note of publications, etc. which have been used, including any agencies which have been employed, and a note of the overall cost and the result: all will prove useful in the long term. Some managers continue to waste money by repeatedly advertising in a selection of publications knowing that one or two of these publications never seem to yield the type of applicants they are looking for. It must be acknowledged that this may be the result of the advertisement itself, that is, it is not attractive enough or it is not pitched at the right level. Alternatively, it could be that the readership of that particular publication does not include the professional group which the manager is trying to recruit from. Whatever the reason, repeated non-productive adverts reflect poor practice.

The question of an attitude towards repeating advertisements which are not initially successful requires careful consideration. The repeated appearance of a post within the same journal may lead readers to believe that here is a hard-to-fill, unattractive post.

If at first an advertisement does not yield a response, and certainly if it does not yield an adequate response on the second occasion, serious consideration should be given to alternative forms of recruitment activity such as the use of other media, a review of the content of the job advertised, or a review of the advertising materials. No one recruitment avenue should be set aside as ineffective until all aspects of the recruitment operation have been reviewed.

The advertising part of recruitment can be said to be complete when the manager has in front of him an adequate number of suitably qualified and experienced applicants to allow the formulation of a short list.

Shortlisting

Shortlisting of applicants for interview should take place against the original 'man specification' for the job rather than against the job description. This follows from the fact that the job description describes the main areas of the job to be undertaken, while the 'man specification' sets out in clear terms the qualities the individual must have in order to carry out the duties associated with the vacant position.

The practice of having long shortlists for a small number of posts or even for one post should be looked upon with some reservation. If the 'man specification' is applied strenuously to each application, then, unless there is an extremely good response towards an advertised post, it is likely that a shortlist of no more than four or at the most five people need be brought forward for interview.

Many managers will be faced with the situation where no one applicant meets completely the specification originally held for the job. When this is the case, a decision must be taken as to whether it would be better to readvertise. It may be that when the market is not likely to yield any better applicants as a result of wider advertising, the manager will be forced to either reduce his 'man specification' or accept that he will not completely fill those requirements. In this case the manager is recruiting in a situation where he must assume that the individual appointed will need time to develop and may require additional training before he can function effectively within the new post.

Once the shortlist has been agreed the final stages of recruitment and selection can now be moved into. In terms of setting up interview times, inviting applicants to attend and conducting the interview, the following points should be borne in mind:

1. Consideration should be given to those applicants who will need to travel long distances.
2. It is necessary to provide suitable times and sitings for interviews; extremely early interviews or interviews late in the day are inconvenient, tiring and will result in candidates and appointment panels not giving their best. Where candidates are travelling some distance, it is good practice to offer to make accommodation arrangements for them and in some cases even travel arrangements may require assistance from the appointing authority in the form of maps and directions for the candidate's use.
3. On writing to the candidates to advise them that they are being invited to attend interview, they should be given clear indication as to where the interview is to take place and at what time. Many employers also like to indicate who the selection panel will consist of and who the other applicants are. It is to the convenience of the candidate to also be given an indication as to whether they will be able to wait and hear the outcome of the interview on the same day or whether they may leave immediately after interview and will be notified by post. Where shortlists are retained to a reasonable length it should be possible to inform candidates before they leave. Keeping candidates (successful and unsuccessful) waiting for notification by telephone or by post cannot be considered good practice. The tension which it involves in the individual can only detract from the good reputation of the employer. Apart from reference to time, place, etc. of the interview, candidates should also be advised of any documentation which they are required to bring with them, for example, evidence of statutory qualifications.

4. It is as well to bear in mind that for many applicants this interview will be their first contact with a particular hospital or authority and that while they may not be suitable for appointment on the day, they may indeed be suitable to apply for another post, so the way in which they are treated on the first occasion becomes very important. Candidates are not likely to return as applicants for a different post, even when invited to do so, if their recollection of that authority on a previous occasion is a poor one.
5. In selecting the interview panel the advice of the National Staff Committee for Nurses and Midwives should always be followed for those appointments which it relates to. Agreement must be reached within the selection panel as to the interview sequence before interviewing starts and particularly in relation to who will cover which areas of the 'man specification' for the appointment. Failure to do this can lead to important areas within the interviewing sequence being left out. This applies whether the interviewers are working to a set 'point plan' or not. Senior managers should ensure that all of their juniors involved in staff selection have received training in interviewing.
6. It is not essential for an interviewing panel to be structured, nor indeed to have a chairperson. However, many people will be more comfortable if the panel is structured and it will be an aid in drawing together the comments of the panel afterwards. It is not usual for outside assessors to chair panels, but it is usual for the panel to consider very carefully the advice which is given by specialist assessors. The employer would be well advised to consider this extremely carefully before moving in opposition. The chairperson, if one is operating, must judge how to manage an interview situation: he may need either to bring a particular line of questioning to a close or to step in and take up points which he feels another individual who was designated that task has not adequately covered.
7. Prolonged arduous interviews are normally an indication of a lack of interviewing expertise or disorganisation within the panel; they do not necessarily indicate thoroughness. The thorough interview is the one which covers each area within the 'man specification' and pursues in detail those points where it seems that the applicant might be weak while at the same time leaving the applicant the opportunity to develop the areas in which they are stronger. Questions which presume or indicate a particular answer should be avoided. An example of this is where a member of the panel asks a question such as: 'Do you like working with groups of people?' This will stimulate most candidates to reply 'yes' because they feel that is what is expected of them. A more open question is desirable.

8. On closure of the interview the interviewees, if they are to wait, should be given some indication of how long they may be kept. This helps them to judge whether or not they are able to get the train they planned to travel on, something which may be a simple, but an important, domestic matter. On completion of the review, and having reached a decision, the chairperson of the panel should always create an opportunity for the unsuccessful candidates to have a short discussion as to why they were not thought to be suitable for the appointment, but only if they wish to do so. This type of post-interview counselling is often best undertaken by the outside assessor, particularly where internal applicants are involved. There are two main reasons for this:
   (a) the assessor can often counsel against a wider professional background; and
   (b) the assessor can do the post-interview counselling without the employee being made to feel that he has failed because of some hidden reason from the past which no-one is telling him about, that is, within his current employment.

Individuals involved in interviewing should bear in mind that when the interview is completed and an offer made to the candidates, the contractual relationship between the applicant and the employer commences. Therefore, the practice of offering a post subject to criteria which are difficult for the would-be employee or the employer to fulfil, or on grounds that are hazy or questionable, should be avoided. When the offer is made, it should be on clear and precise terms and conditions which the applicant can understand.

In terms of the appointment of senior nurses, adequate advice is available from the National Staff Committee for Nurse and Midwives. If adhered to and sensibly applied, the worst pitfalls of interviewing procedure will be avoided.

The ability of management to fill vacancies will stem directly from the availability of applicants and the degree of professionalism displayed by the recruiter.

Training and development

All line managers should be concerned with the training and development of their staff. For the purpose of this chapter, I shall leave aside the question of training for a professional register and concentrate on the type of training and development that is the concern of the line manager in utilising to best effect the manpower which he has available.

It is, unfortunately, often the pattern to undertake training as a response to crisis situations, for example: 'We have no one to do this job!' – 'Ah, train someone'. The other side of the coin is that a number of managers will support members of their staff for attendance at courses which cannot be identified with the needs of the organisation. Some of these difficulties may be avoided by having a training policy which defines the parameter of training.

Where a training policy exists it will normally cover such items as eligibility for course attendance and how to go about obtaining course places, including the important question of authorising attendance. It will describe the benefits available to the applicant including course fees, travel costs, books, etc. It will identify the portion of the training cost to be met by the applicant and where it is all a charge against the authority this will be stated. A training policy can be of great assistance in defining eligibility, who may receive what and indeed encouraging managers to nominate the right people for further training, particularly if eligibility is well defined. It will normally be the decision of the line manager (or in some cases the training department) to nominate and support applicants attending the varying types of training that are available.

Where a manager identifies an individual for further training, this situation is less complicated in terms of a decision to support expenditure on training, as one may presume that the individual identified will in return at least help meet a current service need.

Some employing authorities are in the habit of providing their staff with a prospectus of available courses, some of which will be within their own organisation and others run externally. Such a document requires review each academic year. Where this happens, managers must expect to have their support solicited by staff seeking nomination to the courses available. In attempting to select the individuals for nomination and support, there are a few simple questions which should be posed:

1. Is this type of training relevant to my department? That is, do I require my staff to have the type of skills which they could acquire on such a course? If the answer is 'no', then serious consideration must be given to whether the application is legitimate. The main reason for the employer providing training is in order to meet the needs of the service; there is no duty on the part of the employer to provide for an individual's personal (promotional) development, although, of course, an employer should make provision to train people for the needs of the organisation and for their personal development. Training for the future is one way of meeting the needs of the organisation and developing the individual.

Having accepted that the skills proffered by the course are relevant to the managed department, the next question perhaps is:

2. Is this a reputable course? If not then the applicant can often be guided towards an alternative provision.
3. Finally, is the individual capable of undertaking the course and if so, will he remain in the organisation long enough for the organisation to benefit from its expenditure?

One does not have to look far to find two or three examples of individuals attending expensive courses only to retire two or three months afterwards. The situation leading to such attendances would indeed have to be very special to warrant the outlay of expenditure without return. The manager also needs to consider how the normal duties of the individual are to be covered while they are away for training and how the expenditure is to be met. In short, whenever a request is received for course attendance, the manager must assure himself that the organisation requires the skills which the applicant is seeking to obtain, that he is a suitable individual for the course in question and that the cost and implications can be met.

The training cost will be made up of one or more of the following:

Course related costs:	1. Course Fee
	2. Books
	3. Travel
	4. Subsistence
	5. Typing
Person related costs:	6. Salary and salary on cost
	7. Salary or overtime of replacement
	8. Possible additional study leave (revision or examinations)

The setting of parameters within a training policy will assist the manager in this, but it will never make a decision for him.

It is often the pattern, even where large groups of people are concerned, to send employees outside the organisation on external courses; this happens in terms of management training as well as many other specific skills orientated courses. Often this is the best way to proceed, particularly where the skills to be taught and the necessary resources for teaching them are not available within the organisation. However, there are many situations where training can be conducted 'in house', whether by one's own officers or by tutors brought in from outside organisations. The cost of the 'in house' approach is often more economical, reducing both course costs and the payment of travel and subsistence.

There are further advantages available when considering 'in house' training:

1. It allows greater control over the course organisation and course content.
2. It allows for large groups of people to go through a course at any one time (by reducing costs).
3. Because it is for the employees of one organisation, it can be more easily 'tailored' to local needs and policies.

The main points to consider when deciding on an 'in house' course is whether or not adequate facilities exist locally for mounting courses. This includes resources to undertake the administration of the course and the ability to attract the relevant teaching skills at an acceptable price. If both of these aspects are in the affirmative and there are sufficient candidates, there can be little reason for mounting courses outside of the organisation, other than to assure the mix with individuals from other backgrounds.

It is sometimes the case that managers respond to training departments and colleges by sending pupils only on advertised courses. Training institutions of whatever type expect to respond to the needs of their clients. It is, therefore, often necessary, having ascertained the type of training required, for the client to specify the course content and to ask the institution concerned to mount the course rather than looking down lists of existing courses to find provision which meets with current needs. Failure to adequately clarify one's training needs will lead to institutions providing packaged courses covering what they feel meets the needs of the client but not necessarily the 'real requirement'.

Assessment of training requirements is not always an easy task to complete and it may be necessary to engage some specialist help in order to deal with the preparation of questionnaires and departmental surveys. Any course which is mounted without a considerable amount of thought and some attempt to clarify the needs of the individuals concerned will be less of a success for the individuals; what is more it will be a costly and ineffective matter for the employer.

Different organisations approach the question of managing the budgetary aspects of training in different ways. In the main, there are two approaches. The first is for a department such as a Personnel Department to hold a central training budget. The second is for individual line managers/heads of departments to hold a small budget for training within their departments.

The first allows greater flexibility in spending on training and the latter may inhibit outlay in certain areas and work to reduce the amount of training undertaken by a specific department because of the size of the budget. However, there are cases to be made for both types of budgetary arrangement and in the main, where the department has a large staff requiring a specialised training, it may be best to identify training within the departmental budget. Alternatively in very small departments, and departments only requiring general training facilities, then perhaps it is better if the budget is held centrally. Where this takes place, not only is there more flexibility, but it is also probably easier to control expenditure and gives greater opportunity for training monies to be moved according to changes of emphasis than would be possible within departmental limitations.

Where a department has to undertake regular orientation, induction and in-service training programmes, it may be economical and good practice to consider the use of video equipment. This has the advantage of reducing the amount of personal in-put time required and one is sure that Group B is not having a different presentation to Group A. With the continuing reduction in the cost of video equipment and the wider availability within the NHS, such an approach is now far easier than it was in the 1970s.

Whatever the type of training undertaken, a most important aspect is that of evaluation. All managers engaging outside agencies should insist that an evaluation be undertaken at the end of the course along the lines of a questionnaire or discussion which the nominating officer has helped to design or may take part in. In undertaking course evaluation it is necessary to try and make a clear divide between what the course pupils have enjoyed and what they gain. Not all happy courses are good courses and by the same token not all courses which the participants have not enjoyed are poor courses. Learning can sometimes be painful, particularly when behavioural methods are employed. The real indication of a worthwhile course is the resultant change in performance. Course evaluation should therefore form part of the overall training approach. The evaluation may include the internal 'validation' of the training, that is, a series of tests designed to indicate whether the course has achieved the objectives specified, or external 'validation', that is, a series of tests designed to indicate whether the internal validation relates to the external criteria for the course and the organisational requirements.

Further aspects of evaluation relate to the pre- and post-course performance as seen against the requirements of the organisation. But, unfortunately, it is sometimes the case that none of this is entered into and the only 'evaluation' is a subjective reaction from the participant, which may be affected by events irrespective of the course goals.

Training evaluation in the NHS is further complicated by the lack of 'production' criteria and the presence of subjective criteria, for example, the good of the community.

Apart from reviewing the course content and its effectiveness, it is advisable to annually review all the training that is being undertaken with regard to each department and the whole organisation. Only regular review will identify the need for changes and may lead to more economical and effective ways of undertaking training.

Development of staff on a personal basis will normally come from performance assessment review, although at the same time it may be the organisation's response to a particular developmental wish of an individual. When this is the situation, it should be borne in mind that, as with the correction in deficits of performance, training is not always the answer, and that counselling, advice and alternative experience may all produce the same or a better result. It would also be unrealistic to lose sight of the fact that occasionally one may come across an individual who, in spite of further training, counselling and alternative experience, will not develop in a manner thought desirable by the manager or the organisation.

PERFORMANCE REVIEW

The term 'performance review' as used here indicates the activity of the manager in looking back to establish how an individual has performed in relation to the objectives of the organisation. Within those objectives it is only reasonable to expect that an individual employee, particularly employees in the management grades, will have particular aims set for him during the current management year. To undertake any performance review, whether as part of an organisational review or as part of a formal performance/development review process, would be unfair on the individual if the process did not include target setting.

In setting targets for an individual manager or for a group of staff it is necessary not only to set the targets in terms of what is achievable, but to endeavour to do so with some measure of agreement from those members of staff involved. The target may be in terms of a particular aim, for example, 'introduce a new shift system by October'. Or it may relate to the personal skills (behavioural) aspects of the job, for example, 'develop a more helpful approach to relatives'. Because of the close association between performance and the objectives of the organisation of particular departments, this is a branch of personnel management which of necessity must be undertaken by the line manager; only rarely will assistance by a personnel specialist be required.

Many people have over the years voiced their discontent with the performance review development schemes that have been advocated by National Staff Committees. It may be assumed that part of this is to do with the difficulties that were caused when countersigning officers were removed from the individual employee's work situation, in that they were not normally the people to whom the member of staff reported. In the main, this has now been corrected and forms a sound basis for reviews. However, leaving aside past difficulties of this nature, performance review is not only an important aspect of developing individual members of staff, it is also part of the overall plan of reviewing the effectiveness of the department and to this end must be seen as an ongoing, rather than a once-a-year, process.

Performance review then is not an end in itself, but a means of developing staff and improving the effectiveness of the department in question. It is also a means of raising the department's 'potential' within the organisation.

Where performance review has not been a policy in the past, it may be necessary, depending on the local industrial relations scene, to agree formal performance review procedure with staff organisations. On the other hand, it is not always necessary to have a formal review procedure provided that within the informality the commitment given to the review is meaningful and where action is identified for the future its follow up is not left to chance. Some of the most effective performance reviews, particularly within small departments, are undertaken on the most informal basis.

Where members of staff fail to reach an agreed level of performance, it may sometimes be the case that the inability to realise the target lies with the actual target setting. It is extremely important if individual grievances are to be avoided that the performance standard is attainable in the time given. Where assistance is required from the organisation in order that a member of staff develops new skills, such help should be freely given. Performance assessment and target setting cannot be a one-sided affair. It requires commitment from both the employer and employee.

DISCIPLINE

Disciplinary action is often associated with punishment, whereas the real purpose of discipline is as a last resort in improving performance. While the writer would not suggest there should be any automatic link between performance review and discipline, certainly a persistent failure to reach the required standard of performance can result in disciplinary action, although in practice it is more likely to result from a continued or serious failure to perform to the required standard without targets having been previously set.

The main role, then, of discipline is to improve performance. It is the formalised system employed to warn an individual staff member that his behaviour, that is, performance within the work situation, is not satisfactory and that unless he does something to improve that performance (which may be assisted by management), further formal action will be taken.

The second role of discipline is to protect individual members of the public and in particular patients. It remains linked to the improvement of performance, but occasions do arise where the past actions of the employee are considered to be so serious or detrimental in nature to the public that disciplinary action is taken to protect the public rather than to improve performance of the individual. On no occasion should discipline be viewed as punishment. For this reason the severity of the disciplinary action taken by a manager should relate only to the seriousness with which the organisation views the need to improve performance, not how 'naughty' they feel the individual has been.

Disciplinary activities, like many other activities which are part of the regulation of relationships between the employer and employee, require clear policies and procedures for their operation. As with other policies of this nature affecting employer and employee, they are a matter for negotiation between the host organisation and the staff organisations representing the employees. Following negotiation, it is usual for the policy to be endorsed by the host authority and in the case of the NHS the health authority. From this time on it becomes the formal policy of that authority. This being the case, when a manager proceeds to deal with a disciplinary matter within the policy, he is dealing with it not only as it was negotiated, but as his employer wishes him to deal with it. It is therefore conversely true that where a manager fails to deal with discipline within the agreed policy or for that matter any other subject which is governed by a health authority policy, he is acting outside his employer's wishes, that is, he is not dealing with it in the manner which his employer wishes him to; this being so, he leaves himself open to criticism both from staff organisations and employer, as well as to disciplinary action to correct his own performance!

Disciplinary procedures within the NHS follow a similar pattern. In the main they abide by two principles. First, the principle of natural justice, which in simple terms means that where individuals are likely to have action taken against them which may be to their detriment, it should be done on a fair and equitable basis with the rights of representation and appeal.

Secondly, they are normally constructed within the ACAS code of practice on disciplinary procedures. An example of the procedural part of disciplinary policy is included below.

Procedure

1. Preliminary stage

If an employee's conduct or job performance is in question, the supervisor should investigate the case, and establish the facts before taking any disciplinary measures.

(a) He may find that the employee was not in full control of the events and cannot take full responsibility for the situation. Poor job performance may often be the result of domestic or personal problems or lack of training. In domestic instances, the appropriate course of action would be to hold an informal interview, giving guidance relevant to the circumstances and referring the employee to professional advisory services if necessary. This would normally be carried out by the supervisor or line manager with appropriate advice being given by his superiors and the Personnel Department. If the reason is organisational, appropriate action should be taken.

(b) If it is established that the situation is within the control of the employee, then the supervisor or manager has two alternatives:

(i) *Informal stage*
To give the employee an informal talk in the presence of his appropriate staff representative if the employee so wishes and notify the appropriate line manager. This should be regarded as an opportunity to resolve the matter quickly and quietly. It should be pointed out to the employee the ways in which his conduct warrants disciplinary action and help him to meet requirements in the future; or

(ii) *Formal stage*
If the supervisor feels that an informal warning will serve no useful purpose, then he may pass straight on to the formal procedure stage below:

Note: 'Supervisor' refers to the line manager designated as the employee's immediate superior.

2. Formal procedure

(a) *Admonition – stage I*

The admonition should be given by the appropriate officer of the Health Authority and in the presence of the employee's supervisor, and if the employee so wishes, his appropriate staff representative. The employee should be warned that if his conduct does not improve then he will face a formal warning.

The admonition should be recorded on the employee's personal file and should state the nature of the offence, together with other relevant details, for example, extenuating circumstances.

This admonition may be removed from the personal file after one year if no further written warnings have been issued in respect of the employee's conduct. A period in which to improve may be given to the employee and noted in the file.

(b) *Formal warning – stage II*

If there is no improvement then a formal warning in writing may be given and signed by the appropriate senior officer and it should make clear to the employee that any repetition of the offence or offences will result in dismissal. The warning should be supplemented by a written statement of the facts, specifying clearly the shortcomings of the employee. This should be issued within seven days of the interview and the employee should be informed at the same time of his right of appeal to the Health Authority against the disciplinary action.

A copy of the warning should be kept on the employee's personal file, and if the employee so wishes a copy should be sent to his appropriate staff representative. The warning may include a specified period of time in which to improve, and if the action is successful after 12 months, the record should be cleared other than in exceptional circumstances.

Note: In any cases of improvement periods being given either in Stage I or II, then at the end of the required time the employee should be informed in writing of whether his progress has been satisfactory.

(c) *Dismissal – stage III*

(i) Dismissal (other than in cases of gross misconduct) should only be considered after admonition and formal warning have been issued, and a full investigation of the facts has been undertaken by the appropriate senior officer in consultation with his personnel officer and the appropriate staff representative.

(ii) If, after investigation, dismissal is deemed necessary, then the employee should be given the opportunity to explain his case to his senior officer and his supervisor, and if he so wishes, in the presence of his appropriate staff representative. If the senior officer or employee so wishes, then the Personnel Officer should also be present.

At this interview the employee should again be informed of his right of appeal.

(iii) The dismissal should be confirmed in writing and signed only by the officer with the power of dismissal. Where the employee may only be dismissed by the Health Authority, then the Chairman of the Authority should sign the letter. In this letter the employee should again be informed of his right of appeal.

3. Disciplinary action against a staff representative

If the individual concerned is a union steward or union representative or Professional Association representative, the appropriate full-time officer or professional organisation should be notified before disciplinary action is taken.

4. Summary dismissal

In the most severe cases, for example, theft or violence at work, the responsible manager may wish to carry out immediate dismissal (summary). In the case of gross misconduct leading to immediate dismissal, the manager concerned should, wherever possible, inform the appropriate staff representative prior to formally dismissing the employee. The staff representative should preferably be present when the employee is informed of his dismissal. At this stage the employee must be told that he has a right of appeal against the dismissal. His right of appeal should again be stressed in the letter of dismissal.

When an employee is summarily dismissed, payment will be made up on the last day worked.

The question often arises as to whether or not it is necessary to start at the beginning and work through the whole of a disciplinary procedure, that is, to start with an informal warning, then formal and final warnings before resorting to dismissal. Most policy documents will outline the fact that it is not necessary and will indicate the circumstances under which the manager may miss out one or both of the earlier stages, thereby starting with the final warning. Obviously this must be based on the severity of the incident being dealt with. A common example in terms of nursing is the case of gross misconduct. Such terms as 'gross misconduct' and other expressions that are used to describe a subjectively reached professional decision are often hard to substantiate, particularly at appeal. In specifying the reasons for the disciplinary action, it is desirable to state specifically what is wrong with the individual's performance, rather than simply using expressions like 'gross misconduct', 'failure to reach the required standard', or 'unprofessional conduct'. Clarity can only be given to the situation by quoting the events/incidents which have led to the disciplinary action.

Incidents arise with most professional groups, and certainly in nursing, that should be reported to the professional governing body. In the past this has meant reporting incidents which it is believed put the public, that is, the patient, at risk to the GNC or CMB. The question of reporting an individual to a professional body because it is thought that their activities have caused, or are likely to cause a danger to patients can be separated from the question of disciplinary action by the employer. The reporting of matters to the professional body on the basis of professional concern are not dependent on successful disciplinary action having been taken against the individual. Where cause is given for concern, particularly with regard to the safety of patients, it is necessary to report these instances to the professional body, who, using its own machinery, will make the decision as to whether or not action is warranted. If in doubt, a telephone call to an officer of the professional body concerned will yield help in the form of advice.

There have been instances where actions have been taken in court against members of the profession and where either disciplinary action or reporting the incidents to the registering body concerned have been delayed by the employer until such times as the outcome of the court case is known. In the case of reporting such items to the registering body, this should be done immediately concern is felt; they will pursue their own enquiries and action separately from the court. A finding of 'not guilty' in court does not mean that the registering body will not itself wish to take action to protect the community.

Returning to the question of postponing the employer's disciplinary action until the outcome of the court action is known, this is in the main a poor practice. Awaiting the outcome of court action before taking disciplinary action within the employment situation is a way of abdicating the employer's responsibility to the court. Where the employer has adequate grounds to believe that disciplinary action should be taken in the employment situation, then it is perhaps best if it is done promptly. A finding of 'not guilty' does not mean that the incidents which led to the person appearing in court do not require intervention by the employer on the basis of inadequate or unacceptable performance.

In this sort of case, it is particularly relevant to remember that the facility given to some senior officers to suspend an employee from duty is not part of the disciplinary system nor does it exist with the intention of allowing long-term suspension from duty pending the outcome of the courts. Suspension is a facility to allow an employer to remove the individual from the work situation normally for a very short period while an investigation into an untoward incident or accusation is undertaken. Long periods of suspension, except in rare circumstances where extended or formal enquiries are required, is usually seen as an indication of poor practice. In the majority of cases giving rise for concern, investigation can be completed within a few days, and every attempt should be made to see that this is done and the matter concluded promptly.

There has been a considerable amount of discussion as to whether or not it is right to use a disciplinary procedure as a means of controlling absence and sick leave. While fewer people would argue about the role of discipline in terms of absence (leave taken without permission or certification), the control of sickness by the application of disciplinary procedure is a far more sensitive issue, in so far as part of the performance is a requirement for the individual to be present to undertake the work for which they were engaged. It is reasonable to apply disciplinary procedure to improve an unsatisfactory sickness record even where sickness is certified. However, it has to be noted that for some employees this would be a particularly hard approach.

It would be wrong to give any indication that discipline should be entered into as a means of improving performance allied to non-attendance brought about by ill health until all other approaches had been exhausted. This should certainly include any assistance that can be given in terms of occupational health and possibly an attempt to place the employee in a more suitable line of work where the occupation does not aggravate the condition.

Once embarked on, particularly in cases of chronic long-term illness, the employer may eventually be confronted with the situation where a final warning stage is reached and the individual is still unable to meet the target which the employer has set with regard to return to work. If the employer is not willing to face the inevitability of the dismissal that may result, then discipline should not be embarked upon in the first place. Added to this, it is held by many individuals that there are certain principles which should be adhered to when considering the termination of an employee's occupation on ill health grounds. This includes such considerations as not moving into the dismissal stage with an employee suffering from a chronic condition until such times as they have exhausted their sick pay entitlement. It is also generally held that it is wrong to attempt to terminate an employee's engagement with the authority if they are suffering from a terminal condition.

To summarise on the question of discipline and ill health, disciplinary procedures may be used to correct performance that is inadequate because the individual is irregular at work or away from work for a prolonged period. It is likely to be particularly successful in the case of the odd-day uncertified absences, but can be applied in the case of long-term illness. It should not be applied until all other avenues have been explored and should not lead to termination in cases of chronic ill health where the employee remains in benefit. The writer believes it should not be used in cases of terminal illness.

Comments on monitoring absence and sickness can be found under the heading of 'Manpower Control' below.

HEALTH AND SAFETY AT WORK

The Health and Safety at Work Act 1974 (HASAW Act) and attendant legislation are covered in Chapter 4; for that reason there will be no attempt to cover the legal aspects of Health and Safety at Work in this chapter.

Instead we will look at a number of the management implications of the HASAW Act and indicate the type of action which a manager responsible for a department needs to take in each case. One of the first implications is that the employer must provide a written policy on HASAW. In comparison with some of the other policies agreed in the NHS, this may be more detailed than most people are used to. The Health and Safety at Work policy must be more than a general statement on the subject because of the need to include a statement on how the authority is going to provide for such requirements of the Act as Health and Safety committees, time off for Health and Safety at Work training and the identification of responsible managers.

The majority of organisations will have written this policy a number of years ago and managerial involvement will now be in terms of the following items.

Departmental policy

The presence of an overall policy for the authority does not rule out the need for a departmental policy.

Extract from a general HASAW policy statement

The Authority recognises and accepts its responsibility as an employer under the HASAW Act 1974, for providing a safe and healthy workplace and working environment for its staff.

All reasonable steps will be taken within the resources available to ensure the health and safety of all employees – through training and the provision of maintenance of safe building, equipment and protective clothing.

All managers and supervisors have responsibilities to seek to ensure that adequate provision is made for the health and safety of their staff, and they are trained appropriately, and that safety rules and policy are made known to new employees.

Every employee is reminded that he has a responsibility to safeguard himself and that his own actions, either by instruction, example or behaviour should not put other people or plan or property in jeopardy.

All employees with specific responsibilities for health and safety should ensure that they are adequately delegated in their absence. (This does not necessarily relate to employees in their capacity as safety representatives.)

Adherence to the letter of the law is not sufficient. All staff should work together to make their place of work as safe as possible for patients, visitors and employees. Working routines must be reconsidered regularly to ensure they are safe.

Suggestions are welcome on the elimination of hazards and should be made to the appropriate Head of Department.

Whilst the overall policy responsibility for health and safety rests at the highest management level, individuals at every other level accept degrees of responsibility for carrying out this policy and therefore the Authority will co-operate fully in the appointment of safety representatives. The Authority will consult these representatives on questions of making arrangements to enable the Authority to carry out its duties under the Act, to promote the necessary measures to ensure the health and safety at work of all employees and to check the effectiveness of these measures.

The Authority will also promote measures to ensure that the general public are not exposed to risks to their health and safety.

Contractors working on Authority premises will be required to comply with the working regulations which will be made clear to them when they tender for the work and they must conform to the Authority's safety standards.

This policy may need to be revised in the light of further guidance.

Training

One of the major implications under the Act is the provision of training. This relates not only to making time off available to accredited HASAW Representatives to undertake training, but also refers to the training of new employees in order that they can carry out their duties safely, training to update existing employees, particularly where the task involves changes, plus very specific training, for individuals who work in identified 'potentially dangerous' situations. Add to this the need for management appreciation of responsibilities and of the techniques of audit, and the training investment becomes substantial.

Safe working procedures

The need to write safe working procedures applies to any job undertaken within an organisation which can be identified as having potential dangers to the individual involved. In the nursing field this is often covered by the clinical procedures which seek, as part of assuring good clinical practice, to maintain the safety of the patient and staff. However, more general situations do occur than those covered by the clinical procedures; an example might be working with potentially violent or dangerous individuals as often occurs in mental illness, mental handicap and accident and emergency departments. For this reason, a guidance on the writing of safe working procedures is included below, followed by an example of a safe working procedure.

Writing safe working procedures

In some aspects of employment it is necessary for managers to write and distribute safe working procedures. They are necessary in any situation which may expose staff to risk and should be used as a basis for workplace health and safety education.

Safe working procedures are probably best written at unit level or, where the procedure concerned is specialised or involves a minority group, by the head of department. The type and number of procedures required will vary between places of work. Some managers will need to establish a large number of safe working procedures, while in other areas there will be few.

The purpose of this paper is to provide the basis of a check list whereby those processes that require a safe operating procedure can be identified.

Preliminary check:

1. Are there any Codes of Practice or alternative advice available from authoritative bodies? If so, a Safe Operating Procedure MUST be written and used.
2. Does the general environment situation meet the requirements for heating, lighting and ventilation?
3. Is the work process in itself hazardous because of the system working?
4. Have all the operatives received basic level training which is necessary before they commence work in the department under consideration?

Specific check:

1. Do the operatives work in any of the following situations:
   (a) In confined areas
   (b) Alone
   (c) At heights
   (d) Below ground
   (e) On electrical installations
   (f) On gas installations
   (g) Moving machinery
   (h) With abrasive wheels

(i) In an atmosphere where the process in hand generates dust or other airborne irritants
(j) With violent or disturbed patients
(k) Where there is a lifting content, for example, nursing, stores
(l) Stacking, for example, stores
(m) Handling, for example, loading bays
(n) In extreme temperatures, for example, cold store
(o) In charge of vehicles (safety of loads)

2. Do the operatives work with any of the following:
(a) Infected material
(b) Acids or alkalis
(c) Known carcinogenic agents
(d) Agents likely to give rise to allergies
(e) Volatile or inflammable liquids or gases
(f) Poisons
(g) Steam
(h) Smoke
(i) Boiling water
(j) Boiling fat
3. Do any of the operatives use equipment that is:
(a) Electrical
(b) Gas-powered
(c) Compressed air-powered
(d) Welding, burning, flame-cutting
(e) Abrasive wheels
(f) Dust-creating
(g) Moving (guarded, part-guarded)
(h) Cutting
4. Does the department in question have special requirements in terms of cleaning with regard to:
(a) Procedure
(b) Equipment
(c) Fittings and fixtures
(d) Cleaning of walls, floors and ceilings with special reference to spillage and control of infection, for example, laboratories, wards, kitchens, pharmacy, theatres, etc.

Example of a safe working procedure when handling mercury and amalgam

Mercury vapour is poisonous and may be given off by mercury droplets in the surgery or by waste amalgam. Mercury may be absorbed where vapour is in contact with the skin, not just the hands, and by inhalation. In order to reduce the vapour levels to a safe standard the following procedure must be used:

1. Protect any cut or breaks in the skin before working with amalgam. Avoid wearing open-toed footwear.
2. Place the amalgamator in a well-ventilated area away from a source of heat such as an autoclave/steriliser.
3. (a) Use a 'no touch' technique for handling the amalgam.
   (b) After use wipe the amalgam carrier with spirit.
   (c) Place any disposable material such as spent napkins, contaminated paper tissues and towels or similar items in a lined receiver as soon as possible.
4. Clean instruments free of amalgam before placing in a steriliser.
5. Waste amalgam/mercury must be stored under water in a closed container.
6. Wash hands thoroughly after handling amalgam.
7. Take care to avoid spillage of amalgam or mercury – in order to avoid contamination of bench, floors, shoes, etc. Any spillage must be dealt with promptly. Protect your hands with gloves or plastic bags and use the aspirator to suck up droplets, which may be retrieved from the aspirator bottle. Minute traces may be cleared up with lead foil.

Factory loaded capsules:

1. Do not refill and reuse the capsules.
2. After mixing, open the capsule away from the operator to avoid inhalation of the puff of the mercury vapour which emerges on opening the heated capsule.
3. Immediately replace the cap on the empty capsule and then discard into a lined waste receiver.

Amalgamators/dentomats:

1. The machine should be placed in a drip-tray and be reloaded over this tray.
2. The machine should be adjusted so that it is not necessary to squeeze out the excess mercury from the amalgam mix.

Duty to provide information

Each employer is required to provide for his employees such information as is available with regard to potentially dangerous practices and substances within the field of employment. There are a number of ways of doing this, varying from the well-known 'poster on the wall', handouts, talks and health and safety libraries. Libraries in this context can be anything from a few easily accessible and relevant publications to a full-scale centralised facility.

An important part of protecting the individual from bad practice is by making available to them the information about the potential risks attached to various jobs that they may undertake. In the nursing field, examples of this are handling drugs which could cause allergic reactions, working in x-ray departments and handling infected specimens.

It should be noted that in providing information to employees, it is as important to provide information about good practice as about the areas of risk.

Safety audits

As indicated in Chapter 4, the Health and Safety at Work Act makes provision for safety audits (inspections) to be undertaken following the requisite period of notice by Health and Safety at Work Inspectors. The term 'audit' may be used to include either of these two examples and may also be used to include a check undertaken solely by a manager not accompanied by the Health and Safety Representatives.

As a result of a safety audit, or specific incident or 'near miss', a HASAW representative may issue a hazard notification form. This is a formal notification to management of a 'believed' dangerous or potentially dangerous situation. A brief guide to managers on dealing with hazard notification forms appears below.

Use of hazard notification forms

1. These forms are supplied to Safety Representatives. They are produced in triplicate on self-carbonising paper and consecutively numbered.

   Safety Representatives should complete the form on identifying a particular hazard and send copies, one to the head of department and one to the chairman of the Unit Safety Committee. The third copy should be retained as a record for the safety representative.
2. On receiving the hazard notification form, the head of department should investigate or arrange for an investigation of the hazard to take place.

   He should determine whether he is satisfied that a hazard exists, what remedial action can be taken in the short term, or where appropriate the longer term. A written response must be given on the hazard notification form to the safety representative.

3. The Unit Safety Committee on receiving a copy of the hazard notification form will compile a list to be brought forward at succeeding Safety Committee meetings so that action on these items can be monitored.

Responsibilities of heads of departments

1. Every head of department must have a precise indication of the processes and places of work for which he is responsible. All premises and processes under the control of the Health Authority must have a named manager who is responsible for HASAW aspects.
2. In addition to any management action more routinely taken to investigate the health and safety of the work-place, the head of department must respond to the hazard notification forms.
   (a) Investigate the hazard/potential hazard notified.
   (b) If satisfied the hazard exists, determine what the remedial action should be.
   (c) If this remedial action is long term or costly, consider what short term steps must be taken to minimise the hazard/potential hazard.
   (d) Ensure that staff in the department, the general public, etc. are clearly advised of the hazard and where necessary isolated from it.

Discipline and health and safety at work

A question sometimes arises as to whether or not an individual member of staff can be disciplined for failing to work within health and safety at work policy of the organisation, particularly where they flout safe working procedures to the detriment of other members of staff.

The answer to this is simply 'yes'. Policies are jointly agreed with staff organisations and, as pointed out earlier in this chapter, become the 'rules' of the employing authority. Where a manager believes that an individual is putting himself or others at risk by failing to work in a safe manner, it is reasonable that the disciplinary procedure, if necessary, should be used to correct the practice. The severity of the action taken should obviously match the degree of risk at which the individual is putting himself and others. An example of a severe risk might be smoking in a fuel storage area where it is clear that a 'no smoking' procedure operates. It is not unusual in some industries, for example, where there are large volumes of aircraft fuel stored, for the agreed disciplinary action for an individual found smoking to be a summary dismissal. This is, of course, an extreme example and should not be used as a yardstick for minor failures of performance in the health and safety field.

When the HASAW Act first came into force, it was believed that the amount of time and money that would have to be spent as a result of this legislation would be excessive. There is no doubt that a great deal remains to be actioned for the safety and welfare of employees, but many of the principles of the HASAW Act and the resulting improvement in the safety at work can be achieved by carefulness, training and the inculcation of good practice. Excessive expenditure on the physical aspects of safety is often not the major requirement, but rather good practice.

COMPLAINTS AND STATEMENTS

The question of complaints made by patients, their relatives or others and the taking of statements in connection with the same may be considered a matter of general administration rather than something with personnel management implications. However, because complaints are, in the majority of instances, made against individuals and as the taking of statements can have repercussions on the employer/employee relationship, often with the involvement of staff representatives, it is perhaps reasonable to deal with it as a personnel management matter.

Most Health Authorities will have a local complaints procedure. This is normally written on the basis of dealing with complaints as close as possible to the source and only passing on to the more senior managers those complaints which cannot be adequately dealt with at ward level.

The general approach and procedure for the handling of complaints in the Health Service is outlined in detail in Circular HC(81)5, issued in April 1981. When handling complaints, whatever the source, it is important to impress on members of staff that any individual has a right to complain if they feel they are receiving a less than reasonable service. As soon as words like 'reasonable' are used, the whole matter becomes very subjective and for this reason many complaints are associated with the individual's perception of: (a) what is reasonable, or (b) what may arise from an unrealistic expectancy of what the service is able to provide. Nevertheless, in instances of this nature as with complaints about specific activities, for example, injury to patients, loss of clothing, missing money, the complainant has a right to complain and NHS officers have the duty to investigate.

Some local complaints procedures require the complainant to put the complaint in writing. From the point of view of retaining on record a clear statement of the complaint, this is a good idea. The failure of an individual to 'write down' his complaint does not in any way reduce the seriousness with which the complaint can be viewed. Complaints made verbally may be just as serious as those made in writing and as such should be investigated in the same way. It is not unheard of for a member of the public to 'mention' something to a member of staff and finish the discussion by saying: 'I don't really want to complain – I'll leave it with you to do whatever you think is right.' In these circumstances, I have always found it safer if the member of staff makes a record of the conversation, presuming the complainee will not; it can then be treated as any other complaint. Failure to do so leaves both that particular member of staff and the whole of the organisation open to criticism at a later date. In short, the individual officer does not have any discretion in the matter of filing complaints and their investigation. When a complaint is made, however it is made, it must be investigated in a thorough and sensitive manner and the outcome of that investigation made known to the complainant. In this way the record is straight from the beginning and the service cannot be accused of trying to hide anything. The complainant, if unsatisfied with the outcome, can take the matter to a higher level of authority for investigation and eventually if still dissatisfied to the Ombudsman.

In seeking to take statements from staff whether it be in connection with a complaint or an untoward incident, it is perhaps necessary to establish the difference between seeking a report and asking the individual to make a statement. The line between the two is extremely thin and very difficult to define. It is, however, important to understand that when a member of staff is asked within their normal duties to provide information about work-related matters, verbally or in writing, it is reasonable that they do so. Failure to undertake the report required may result in the employer taking action against them if persuasion and discussion fails to obtain the required information. The grounds for this are that the individual employee has refused a reasonable management request.

Making a statement, on the other hand, although very hard to separate from report-writing, tends to infer that the individual is in a position where they feel threatened, for example, they have been involved in an untoward incident, something has gone wrong with the administration of drugs and they feel that they may be held responsible, or where a member of staff is being investigated with regard to complaints of theft. Here, understandably, the individual may feel that they will be disadvantaged by making a statement and for this reason may wish to: (a) refuse; (b) have a little time to prepare their statement; (c) take advice before doing so. All of these actions are reasonable and should be encouraged by the manager requesting the statement, providing undue delays are not incurred. In the case of the individual refusing a statement because he feels threatened, it must be understood that this is the individual's right and if he cannot be persuaded to make a statement, then he should not be coerced into doing so.

Individuals can be helped in writing statements if they are encouraged to use the following principles:

1. An indication as to why the individual is providing the statement.
2. If a statement refers to a particular incident, the individual should, as far as possible, indicate the date and the time when the incident took place and anyone else who was present at the time.
3. He should try to record the events as they happened, that is, in chronological order.
4. The information that appears in the statement should be only that which he knows to be certain rather than hearsay or the expression of opinions.

The statement should be signed at the end, dated and the individual encouraged to keep a copy. The poor quality of statement is sometimes related to lack of facilities for typing, etc. The investigating manager can often be of assistance in this area.

While individuals may decline to give a statement, it should be pointed out to them that, if at a later date they are required to attend an enquiry, or indeed if the matter should be of interest to the courts, their position might in fact be worsened by not having made a statement at the time. This is partly because their memory will not be good as to the detail of an incident two or three years later and partly because a court may only admit as evidence a statement made soon after the incident. Also in the case of a court hearing the nurse who has not previously made a statement may be deprived of any 'note' to refer to if called as a witness. Where statements are subject to question at a later date, particularly in court, it will assist the individual in speaking to his original statement if he has kept to those matters which he knows to be so, has avoided flowery phrases and expressions open to misinterpretation and has refrained from drawing conclusions which might at a later date prove erroneous – in short, he should be truthful, concise and clear.

DISCRIMINATION

'Discrimination' in employment terms has in the main come to mean discriminating against an individual, usually on the basis of his sex, race or religion and it is this type of discrimination which the present legislation seeks to remove, although other types of discrimination are not unknown. There are many ways in which an employer can intentionally or unintentionally discriminate against an individual or group of individuals, but it is most likely to happen in terms of the appointment of staff or the selection of staff for training and promotion.

Many managers have on occasions felt that they could be criticised when, during their normal selection procedure, they have declined to appoint an individual from a minority group. There is no reason for managers to be concerned in this way providing they have applied the selection procedure fairly. This is another reason why it is so important to review job descriptions and to write 'man specifications' before appointment procedures begin. If this is done then it will be easy to show what the criteria for the post were and how an individual applicant did or did not meet those criteria. To put this argument another way round, it is fair to turn down an applicant for appointment if they do not meet the specification for the job, but at the same time the specification for the job must be realistic for the work to be undertaken. Some examples of this are as follows:

1. If a manager turns down a lightly built female who has applied for a post on the ground that she is not strong enough, it is very likely that this would be seen as discriminatory, unless the real requirement of the job was that they should be able, for example, to lift certain weights. If the job specification stated 'must be able to lift 140lb unaided', then it would be expected that the manager would take steps during a selection procedure to assure himself that an individual could lift a weight of 140lb unaided, but even then it is only an acceptable criterion if a part of the job actually requires the individual to undertake that type of task. It should not be put there just to exclude the lighter-built women.
2. If a requirement for a post is that the successful applicant must have 'A' level mathematics, that may be quite fair and reasonable if, for example, the job requires a mathematical ability to 'A' level standard. To place that requirement into a 'man specification' purely to rule out a racial group which has not had the educational opportunities to do 'A' level maths would be discriminatory. So having placed the requirement within the 'man specification', the manager must feel comfortable that it is a real requirement.

The paragraphs above may suggest a rather negative approach to avoiding discrimination. While this is not intentional, perhaps a better approach is to indicate the more positive ways of avoiding discrimination. The first step is for the employer to declare a policy of 'equal opportunities'. Any such policy must acknowledge and work within the legal background. This is referred to in the Sex Discrimination Act 1975, the Race Relations Act 1976 and the Trade Unions and Labour Relations Act 1974/76. Where discrimination occurs on the basis of race, colour, sex/'marital' status or trade union membership, individuals have a right of access to the Industrial Courts to seek redress. An excerpt from a policy which states an employer's intention to provide equal opportunities is given below:

Statement of policy

This document states Policy of the Health Authority that all its employees will be given an equal opportunity in matters relating to their employment. No employee or job applicant should receive less favourable treatment in recruitment, terms and conditions of service or dismissal on the grounds of race, colour, ethnic or national origin, religion or creed, trade union membership, a spent criminal conviction, pregnancy, sex, homosexuality, marital status or on the grounds of disability.

Selection, promotion, treatment and training must therefore be on the basis of relevant merits and abilities without conditions or requirements which cannot be shown to be justifiable. The Authority expects its officers not merely to avoid discrimination but to develop positive policies to promote equal opportunities in employment.

Positive policies to promote equal opportunity may include the provision of crèche facilities and flexi-hours, although the latter is not usually possible in nursing.

In terms of a manager's check list of action to avoid discrimination the following may be useful:

1. review the criteria used for recruitment, training and promotion decisions to ensure that all are essential and relevant to the job;
2. review all documents such as advertisement, job descriptions, etc. to establish that there are no discriminatory practices or job titles;
3. discuss with your subordinate managers/supervisors the arrangements for recruitment, training and promotion in their departments.

Any member of staff is entitled to his opinions on discrimination. It is often an emotive issue but opinions are all that he is entitled to. He must act within the legislation and principles mentioned; to do otherwise is illegal.

MANPOWER CONTROL

Many people reading this will expect to see a section on manpower planning. It has been avoided because the writer believes that the most pressing question for junior and middle line managers is manpower control. However, those wishing to gain information on the subject of manpower planning will find a large number of references available in the DHSS publication entitled *Nursing Manpower – Maintaining the Balance* (March 1982).

The ability to control manpower is perhaps the most important aspect of the line manager's personnel management activities. It does not mean so much controlling in terms of 'making people do as they are told', but in ensuring that man hours are not wasted.

To practise 'manpower control' means having available adequate information about the structure of the workforce that is being managed, its weaknesses and its strengths, including information about experience and qualifications and, in particular, time lost. Manpower control as a concept presumes that managers will take informed decisions about employment practices on the basis of manpower information. One major area of this is the control of absence and sickness. It would be wrong to give the impression that the only aspect of control applicable to absence and sickness is the application of the disciplinary procedure, and attention has already been drawn to the health aspect of controlling lost hours through sickness. Before any form of control can be exerted and particularly in the case of time out (an expression used to include any time lost from the working environment), adequate information must be obtained about the actual time out. This can be done on a local basis, using card record systems or it can be done using the medium of microcomputers to record absences of all types. Alternatively, it can be undertaken on larger computer systems fed via the salaries and wages input, as is the case with the standard payroll system (SPS) and its relationship to the Standard Manpower and Planning Personnel Information System (STAMP).

An exceptionally large amount of data is already available within the NHS regarding the staff employed. This includes information of a personal nature, for example, name, address, age, sex, qualifications, data regarding time lost, shift patterns, number of staff employed in particular places and at particular times, the relationship between the number of staff and the number of patients, as well as data on patterns of hospital activity, when the admission rates to medical wards rise and fall, which days are the busiest, which nights of the week are the busiest in accident and emergency departments, etc. It is taking this data and turning it into useful information on which management decisions can be based about the way that we can use our staff which is so important.

Let us look at some of the systems at present in use to convert some of that data into useful information.

STAMP

While predominantly a planning information system, much of the data available on STAMP is useful for control purposes as well. The major drawback in using this system as a control system is allied to it being a 'batch' system and the weaknesses outlined below:

Excerpt from STAMP handbook – Oxford Regional Health Authority

DESCRIPTION OF THE STAMP SYSTEM

The basic STAMP system extracts information from weekly and monthly payroll files and sorts and stores this in the form of a magnetic tape record for each individual employee. The main record is a large and complex file containing all the information listed in Appendix 6.1 for current employees and leavers since 1 April each year. A tape is kept for each financial year so that it will be possible to look back on past employees' records. A historical record is kept for current employees giving details of promotion and transfers, etc.

Most of this information is derived from SPS (Standard Payroll System) computer files. It follows that the accuracy of STAMP information is only as good as the accuracy of payroll input. Payroll managers have the responsibility for paying staff correctly and the input of information required to do this (grade, hours, allowances, deductions) is likely to be of a high standard. For other details which are input primarily for information purposes (for example, birth date, occupation, code, unit code) payroll managers depend on personnel officers and line managers feeding in the correct information. It is therefore the responsibility of all officers who are involved in the recruitment and payment of staff to ensure that the data contained in SPS and STAMP files is as accurate and up to date as possible.

Not all manpower information required by managers is available in payroll files. STAMP makes provision for the addition of information on date of start in NHS; nationality; ethnic origin and historical data on current employees. Such information can be input to STAMP using a special form. The input of further information (for example, absence, qualifications) will have to await further development of the STAMP system.

INFORMATION OUTPUTS

The system provides four main practical ways of obtaining printouts.

1. Standard printouts:
   Routinely produced at monthly or longer intervals and covering all staff.
   These are:
   Title
   Nominal roll
   Hour analysis
   Headcount by financial code
   Headcount – district summary

Starters and leavers (turnover) analysis
Age analysis
Retirement schedule

In addition there are two standard printouts not routinely produced:
Master file (individual) print
Cost analysis print

Detailed information on the coding system used in STAMP, in future developments and special facilities, for example, 'Design a form' for special searches, is available from Regional Health Authorities using STAMP, normally in the form of a handbook or manager's guide.

STAMP is not available in all Health Regions and this has led to some authorities solving their manpower information needs by the installation of local systems or the use of computer bureau services.

SNIPPET

One example of a computer bureau service is the SNIPPET system developed for nursing in certain districts of the North Western Region in conjunction with ADP Network Services. SNIPPET – Standard Nursing Information Package for Planning Evaluation and Training – covers in four modules, personnel, GNC management and financial control related data. The last of these remains under development (at September 1982) and will involve the transfer of data from the Standard Payroll System concerning hours of duty and overtime costs to the employee. This is a nursing information system.

NHPPD

The availability of information for manpower control purposes does not have to relate to computerised systems. The use of dependency studies related to staff availability is equally important. Much has been written on dependency which is available in nursing libraries but a simple-to-use tool which may be of use to managers wishing to look at 'actual' staffing in relation to patients after all time out is deducted is the 'Nursing Hours Per Patient Day' approach. This easy-to-use-technique, which was developed in the Oxford Region, uses staffing rotas and patient occupancy figures to arrive at an assessment of time available per patient. The study may be done by day or night, NHPPD or NHPPN, and can be calculated for any grade or group of nursing staff and for any ward or group of wards. In practice, it is often convenient to classify the staff into trained (SRN and SEN), learners (students and pupils), and others (nursing auxiliaries, etc.). Since night cover is generally low, grouping into trained and total staff is usually appropriate.

The midnight count of patients may seem an inadequate representation of the ward activity during the daytime. Other indices could be formed from the data, such as the addition of the number of admissions and discharges to the bed occupancy. In the final analysis, however, the index is no more than an exploratory tool which serves to highlight differences in the current deployment of nursing staff. While some of these differences are due to variation in the type of patient and/or prescribed treatment régimes, there are many instances where the ratios for similar wards are markedly different and cannot be readily explained. Where this occurs, further studies are essential to establish both the cause and effect. Details of the NHPPD approach are available from the Nursing Department, Oxford Regional Health Authority.

Manpower control relies then on the availability of reliable information and on a system of data capture. All are tools; the decision-making remains with the manager but can be aided by a well-thought-out system of data capture and information presentation.

NEW TECHNOLOGY

In the 1970s, perhaps one of the major challenges to nurse managers was the changing pattern in the industrial relations scene brought about by changes in legislation and a new awareness of nurses in trade union activity. While some organisations still struggle with industrial relations problems, the majority have now passed through the period of stabilisation into calmer waters.

What then of the future? Change will always be present in nursing; some of it will be major and will call for changes of work practice and training. One such area currently acting upon the profession is the field of technology.

There are only a handful of Health Authorities in the UK that have already experienced changes in nursing as a result of the installation of computers and associated gadgetry. For the rest, it is a development to be looked forward to both with excitement and trepidation.

While there are many benefits to be reaped, particularly from computerised systems relating to health care, there are also many implications for employment practice which will require action in the personnel management field. If the majority of hospitals and in particular District General Hospitals are to follow the 'few' – as they must – in computerising patient master indexes, admissions and discharges, waiting lists, out-patient appointments and many aspects of ward ordering, to mention only a few areas of activity, they must be careful to involve nurses.

Presuming the involvement of nurses in identifying the information needs of authorities and the operational systems which will meet these needs, the second major area of activity will be in establishing policy on the introduction of new technology, training staff and continually reviewing nursing needs and practices in line with developments. Systems which provide for the needs of the information gatherers yet do not assist the delivery of care should be avoided.

There are a number of ways of approaching policy on new technology but once the general policy has been established then the policy on its introduction must be dealt with. Reaching agreement with the staff organisations concerned is likely to be an area for local negotiation for some time to come and as such will produce a policy which hopefully meets the needs and realises concerns of the staff organisations but allows the introduction of new technology to move ahead.

Some employers will seek to have one agreement on the introduction of new technology covering all groups of staff in all departments; others will opt for agreements to cover specific departments or applications. The latter is perhaps the easiest to manage as the conditions of the agreement can be related to a known application (hardware and software). General agreements tend to be either very long and unwieldy or so general as to be negative. Agreements by departments are useful where applications are restricted to one group of staff but are usually only possible in specialist situations, for example, haematology.

There is a considerable amount of information available on new technology agreements from trade unions and in management handbooks, but in the main the agreement should deal with the following:

1. Information on the proposed system, including type of hardware and software, the job it will do and its effect on work practice.
2. Provision for consultation on working arrangements, skill requirements, job numbers and levels plus working conditions.
3. Provision for a statement on health and safety allied to the proposed system.
4. Provision for a statement on retrieving and redeployment of skill where applicable.
5. Arrangement for handling the negotiation of an agreement, its amendment or termination.

The training implication of introducing computers to the health care situation can, for nurses, be divided into categories, presuming that the 'technical' management of the system will be undertaken by non-nurses:

1. Orientation to Health Service computing.
2. Introduction to the proposed system.
3. 'Hands on' training for operators.
4. Updating on system changes and replacement training of new staff.

Because of the size of the nursing workforce, any system which involves all nursing staff, for example, nursing orders system in a district general hospital, it is likely that the only realistic approach to training will be by 'cascade' principles, the tutors and nursing officers being trained to a higher level in advance so that they may form the 'core trainers'. For this reason, training costs are more likely to be in terms of manhours than course fees as the terminals in wards, etc. can be used for on-the-job training. Nevertheless, such training is a major commitment which needs to be budgeted for. The following might be seen as a very rough guide to the size of the commitment in a hospital with 900 nurses:

Core training:
30 nursing officers and ward sisters @ minimum of 20 hours each
= 600 hours

870 nurses @ minimum of 3 hours each = 2,610 hours

Total Minimum Training Time = 3,210 manhours

Added to this is repeat time for those nurses who progress more slowly and the replacement of any 'core trainers' who may leave. Some time must then be allocated each year for system and staff changes.

But if it could be done in 3,210 hours at an average cost of only £2.50 per hour, the implied cash cost presuming no overtime rate, that is, all flat rate replacement, is £8,025. On top of this would be the cost of any films, videos, handouts and machines!

Training and its allied problems must not be allowed to slow down the advance of nursing into computerisation. If we allow this to happen, we will delay the arrival of reliable management information, better use of nursing resources, the reduction of consumables, waste and 'clerical tasks' for many years, and at the same time place nursing in the position of accepting what others have to offer rather than what nursing requires.

POSTSCRIPT: A DEVELOPMENT IN MANPOWER CONTROL

During the time that this publication was being prepared for print, the Government of the day introduced a new, and many would say ill-conceived, method of controlling manpower in the National Health Service. This initiative by central Government brought into being the concept of manpower targets as a control mechanism. Readers wishing to see the 'formal' statement on this will find it in the DHSS Health Circular HC(83)16.

Traditionally, the only central Government control over the number of staff employed in the service had been through the operation of cash limits. In short, this meant that if you had the revenue to pay staff at Regional or Health Authority level you might do so. There was no control of the number or discipline of staff recruited.

HC(83)16 brought cash limits and manpower targets into the same arena; here lies the reason for the claim that the concept of limiting the number of people to be employed is ill conceived. For to limit both cash and manpower by separate mechanisms in an industry where manpower is the major expenditure is, to say the least, 'odd'.

What could have led to this situation? It has been claimed that because the Health Service failed to respond to a request from the Government to set manpower targets and because there was an increase in manpower across the board during a period of 'no growth', central action was considered necessary.

The action required as a result of the issue of HC(83)16 meant that health Regions were faced with making plans to reduce the numbers of staff employed by 1 per cent overall. For this purpose the Government departments divided staff in two categories; the first including doctors, dentists and nurses (professional and technical) was to bear a 0.75 per cent to 1 per cent reduction, and the second, a reduction of between 1.35 per cent and 1.8 per cent.

The rationale for this lay in the argument that in the unexpected increase of staff prior to 1983, the increase in non-professional staff had been disproportionate to the increase in professional staff.

Many of the problems which arose from this approach and are consequently suffered by the Service are born out of the following dilemmas.

First, regions had to agree a 31 March 1983 base line against which the reductions could be made. As the DHSS figures were based on a Census tape (snap shot) taken at 30 September 1982, the 31 March 1983 base line was only an estimate resulting from reconciliation with the 30 September 1982 Census which was subject to Government agreement. Only in this basis could the 31 March 1984 target be set (the date by which reductions must be achieved).

Secondly, having reached this point, how were Regions to divide the reduction (cuts) between Health Authorities? Many different mechanisms were used and below are some of the options:

1. To establish a District Authority's target based on:
   - Ratio of staff to population served
   - Reduction pro rata to total staff employed
   - Reduction pro rata to staff employed in hospitals at 31 March 1983
   - Reduction pro rata to staff employed in acute service
2. To use weighted options; there were a number of these including staff to available acute beds, staff to discharges and deaths, etc.
3. To base the reductions on the Authority's distance from sub-regional RAWP targets
4. To use a subjective sliding scale on the basis of 'achievement'.

Each of these brings its own problems even before the division of the targets between professional and non-professional staff.

Following the agreement of targets to be met by 31 March 1984, the Secretary of State for Social Services agreed that in the next round of target setting (1984) the division between the two staff groups would be removed, thereby giving Authorities more flexibility in operating the continuing method of manpower control. It is likely that when this book is published, 'manpower targets' will still be in force; if so, what are the future implications for nurse managers?

There are many, but I will suggest only three here:

1. Nursing will no longer be protected from taking a larger cut than other staff groups because of the 1984 'flexibility'.
2. New projects will have a better chance of success in that they have low manpower implications.
3. Any new project that by the recruitment of additional manpower pushes the Regional figures over the 'target' level is likely to require Government approval.

Is there a way round this untidy mechanism? Well, there are ways of living with it and they are all to do with priorities and good man management. But round it, no! Certainly not by paying overtime because then the manager falls on the other prong of the HC(83)16 fork: it is called 'cash limits'.

Suggested further reading

Austey, E. (1977) *An Introduction to Selection Interviewing*. London: HMSO.

Code of Practice for Prevention of Infection in Clinical Laboratories and Post Mortem Rooms. London: HMSO.

DHSS (1981) *Circular HC(81)5.*

Health & Safety – Notification of Accidents and Dangerous Occurrences. Regulation 1980.

Health & Safety at Work – Safety Representatives and Safety Committees. London: HMSO.

Nursing Manpower – Maintaining the Balance (1982) DHSS.

Randall, G.A., Packard, P.M.A., Shaw, R.L. & Slater, A.J. *Staff Appraisal.* London: Institute of Personnel Management.

Chapter 7
Managing Finance

DAVID MOSS

THE FINANCING OF THE NATIONAL HEALTH SERVICE

The level of spending on the NHS

The Royal Commission of 1979 reported that since 1949 total expenditure on the NHS had more than doubled in real terms and that the value of resources devoted to the NHS had increased in every year except 1952. Total expenditure had grown faster than the rest of the economy in almost every year since 1954, rising from 3.4 per cent of the gross domestic product (GDP) in 1954 to 5.6 per cent in 1977. In 1983/84 the Government plan to spend £13,000 million on the NHS.

The Royal Commission also made international comparisons and concluded that although many other developed countries devote a higher proportion of their GDP to health care than the UK, there is no evidence that this leads to an improved health status for their populations. Moreover, there is clear evidence that whatever expenditure is incurred on health care, the demand for health care will always tend to grow faster than the supply.

The method of financing the NHS

It is important to remember that the NHS is almost wholly funded by the Exchequer. The source of funds is approximately as follows:

General taxation 88%
National insurance 9%
Income from charges 3%

The method of financing the NHS obviously exerts an important influence over its financial management but it does not mean that its financial problems are in any way unique. Other countries with quite different financing mechanisms are wrestling with the same problems of controlling expenditure and achieving value for money.

In the end, both the level of spending and the method of financing health services are matters of political choice and form part of the overall debate about the desirable level of public expenditure or private enterprise and about the relative priority of health as against other types of public or private expenditure. Most managers in the NHS will argue that more health care expenditure is desirable but, ironically, few are confident that the whole of the existing expenditure is either necessary or desirable.

THE FINANCIAL ALLOCATION MECHANISM

Determination of overall public expenditure levels and the balance of priorities between programmes

The Government of the day clearly has the duty to set the overall level of public expenditure and determine the overall allocations between spending departments.

The planning mechanism for public expenditure is known as PESC (Public Expenditure Survey Committee). This committee formulates detailed proposals for the Chancellor of the Exchequer to debate in Cabinet. An annual public expenditure White Paper then emerges which sets out the Government's expenditure forecast for the next three years.

The White Paper is a forecast, not a control mechanism. The control mechanism is the parliamentary estimates which are voted each year and which form a basis of control of the NHS spending at a national level in the DHSS.

Resource allocation at national level – allocations from the DHSS to the Regional Health Authorities

Revenue

Revenue expenditure is defined basically as day-to-day expenditure on ongoing services. The equity of resource allocation is one of the most vexed questions of financial management in the NHS. The original NHS Act (1946) enshrined the objective of a national service uniformly available on the basis of need. Nevertheless, on the basis of expenditure per head of population, a palpable mal-distribution has continued and developed in the NHS. The most serious effort to tackle this problem was the Resource Allocation Working Party (RAWP) which reported in 1976 and whose recommendations strongly influence the DHSS allocations to Regional Health Authorities since that date.

The RAWP formula for revenue distribution seeks to allocate resources on the basis of overall measure of need. The formula uses population weighted by age and sex as the basic measure of need. The population measured is also weighted by the standardised mortality ratio (as proxy for morbidity) and adjusted for cross-boundary flows. Separate allowance is made for London weighting and the extra costs of teaching (through SIFT, the Service Increment for Teaching).

The calculation of an overall weighted population is then used to compute a Regional Target allocation in relation to the overall funds available. Actual allocations are then compared with targets to establish relative over- and under-provision.

A key issue arising from this approach is the question of whether at Regional level resources should be removed from over-provided Regions (over-target Regions) to be transferred to the under-provided Regions or whether differential growth funds should be allocated in order to gradually raise the relative level of funding in the poorer Regions. So far the latter course has generally been pursued by governments (for example, with the revised national growth of 1.3 per cent in 1982/83, the North West Thames Region received 0.2 per cent whereas the East Anglia Region received 2.6 per cent). Under this method, pace of movement towards equity will be painfully slow and may be non-existent if the overall growth in the NHS reduces or ceases altogether. In 1983/84 the national growth rate was only 0.2 per cent and for the first time some Regions had a negative growth rate of up to 0.7 per cent while the maximum positive growth was 1.9 per cent.

Capital

Capital is basically defined as expenditure on the acquisition of assets. The capital RAWP mechanism is similar to revenue in that targets of capital stock have been computed by relating actual capital stock to the weighted population of each Region. Actual capital stock has been defined as stock in existence in 1961 valued at estimated replacement cost plus actual capital expenditure since 1961.

In implementing capital RAWP, the DHSS has earmarked capital to some individual major schemes and has distributed the balance of the capital allocation in relation to RAWP targets but on a very phased basis to avoid rapid decreases or increases in the capital programmes of individual regions.

Joint finance

Joint finance is an earmarked allocation (which can be spent on revenue or capital) for schemes jointly agreed between Health and Local Authorities.

The schemes can cover the field of primary care, social services, education for the disabled and housing.

Joint finance is intended as a stimulus to collaboration between Health and Local Authorities on services of mutual interest, especially services for the disabled, the elderly, the mentally ill and the mentally handicapped.

The distribution of funds from the DHSS to Regions is based on population served weighted to take account of:

1. population aged over 75;
2. the use of health facilities by the mentally ill and mentally handicapped;
3. the incidence of inner city populations.

It should also be noted that joint finance is a pump priming allocation. It can meet all or part of capital costs but revenue costs have eventually to be picked up on a phase basis by the Local Authority or the Health Authority.

Resource allocation within regions – allocations from the Regional Health Authorities to the District Health Authorities

Revenue

Regional Health Authorities have the duty of allocating finance for activities at Regional level and to their constituent District Health Authorities (DHAs). Finance will therefore be earmarked for the costs for the Regional Headquarters and for any Regionally managed services (for example, computers, blood transfusion). Some Regions charge out Regionally managed services to District Health Authorities and therefore do not hold a central allocation.

With regard to the funding of Regional clinical services – certain specialised services are recognised as being Regional specialties and therefore receive special funding recognition. Mechanisms vary between Regions but the general principle is that the funding of these services is excluded from the calculation of the main funding formula for DHAs.

Nurse managers should be familiar with the funding policy of their Region and be prepared to critically appraise its implications for nursing services. Many Regions operate a form of RAWP allocation whereby revenue resources are gradually being moved towards Districts that are underfunded in proportion to their weighted population. Some Regions have been far more radical than others in seeking to achieve a genuine redistribution of resources.

Some Regions have perpetuated the funding of revenue consequences of capital schemes (RCCS) to Districts. This may be a convenient way of avoiding the failure to open new buildings but it tends to be highly retrogressive in terms of achieving equitable distribution of resources. It also has the effect of shifting resources towards the acute sector with its expensive capital infrastructure and away from the more community-based services for the mentally ill, handicapped and the elderly. Nurse managers should press for a Regional funding policy which gives proper recognition to their District in terms of the needs of their population.

Capital

Most Regions hold a large part of the capital allocation at Regional level in order to finance central management of capital schemes. Regions are generally attempting to assess the relative distribution of capital within Regions in order to move to a more explicit longer-term allocation policy in relation to each DHA.

Regions do delegate some capital schemes to DHAs and also make minor capital allocations on a formula basis. It is for DHAs to decide the use of the minor capital allocation.

Nurse managers should take a much stronger interest in the allocation and management of capital. Capital is the agent of change in the character of service provision in many parts of the service and nurses should press for greater delegation. Some capital schemes are unnecessarily expensive and therefore the service is deprived of other possible developments. Nurses should also use their influence to achieve a proper balance between capital and revenue investment.

Joint finance

Regions are free to vary the national formula in allocating joint finance to DHAs providing proper weighting is given to the population served by services for the elderly, mentally ill and mentally handicapped. Some Regional earmarking takes place and in general funds are allocated to DHAs on a formula basis.

Joint finance can provide a major opportunity for innovative community-based initiatives. Nurse managers should therefore find out how the allocation mechanism works in their DHA/Region.

Nurse training schools

The financing of nurse training schools is outside the national process for the distribution of revenue, capital and joint finance (nurse managers may be relieved to know). The DHSS allocates funds to the English National Board which in turn distributes it to the Schools of Nursing on the advice of the Regional Interim Education Advisory Groups. However, the cost of students and pupils falls on the main Health Authority budget.

The funding of inflation

The rate of pay and price increases and the Government's policy on the funding of these increases are among the most critical issues faced by Health Authorities and their managers. In the days when allocations were subject to an annual retrospective revaluation based on actual pay and price increases, inflation tended to be viewed as something that happened outside the Health Service. *This is no longer the case.* It is important to realise that the Health Service is now funded according to a Government forecast of expected (or desirable) inflation. A pay award above the cash limit provision can, therefore, wipe out growth funds. Similarly, a drop in the rate of price increases below the Government forecast can give Health Authorities a financial bonus and can stimulate real growth in the Service. Treasurers calculate the detailed implications of expected and actual pay awards and monitor movements on the Health Service Price Index, which measures the changes in prices of expenditure relevant to Health Services. They should advise managers frequently of the effect of these trends.

THE FINANCIAL ACCOUNTABILITY MECHANISM

The management of services within cash limits

Health Authorities have a statutory duty not to overspend their cash limits in a particular financial year. In any case, on revenue all overspendings are carried forward as a reduction on the allocation in the following financial year. Health Authorities may carry revenue underspendings of up to 1 per cent forward to the next financial year (any greater underspending is lost). Similar rules operate for capital. In addition, Health Authorities can transfer up to 1 per cent of revenue to capital and up to 10 per cent of capital to revenue. They have no power to borrow or lend money along the lines operated by Local Authorities.

The definition of cash limits and income and expenditure

Cash limits are defined (in summary) as cash advances for local payments plus central payments (tax and national insurance (NI)) plus non-cash transfers (for example, superannuation and centrally purchased supplies). Authorities, after taking account of the locally generated income, requisition cash to meet charges on their cash limits. The national system of public expenditure control works on a cash receipts and payments basis and from the point of view of Parliament and the Treasury, a prime duty of the treasurer is to ensure that his Authority operates within its cash limit. Although nurse managers should be interested in cash flow, their primary concern as budget managers will be with control of income and expenditure. There is an important distinction between income and expenditure accounting which measures actual consumption of resources and cash limits which reflect the cash drawings. There will clearly be a difference between cash drawn and expenditure incurred (for example, changes in balances such as debtors, stocks and creditors).

The statutory accounts

One method of formal accountability is the production of the annual accounts and cost statements. The annual accounts summarise the financial performance of the Health Authority in terms of both income and expenditure and charges against cash limits. They also contain a balance sheet and a statement of source and application of funds. They are the key mechanisms for the DHSS to account to Parliament for NHS expenditure by producing the national Appropriation Account. However, the annual accounts are of little use to nurse managers as a management tool.

The cost statements will be of more interest to nurse managers. These statements currently analyse expenditure for each hospital on a departmental functional basis (the primary analysis) and between in-patients, out-patients, accident and emergency cases, day cases, day patients and other patients (the secondary analysis). Unit costs per case, per in-patient day, per out-patient day, etc. are also produced, which make possible comparisons between hospitals of the same type. Supplementary cost statements are produced for a number of functions, for example, estate management, catering, radiography. There are also separate cost statements for community and ambulance services. Community health service accounts have the same functional analysis as hospital services, but have a secondary analysis of expenditure between school health services, general community care (clinics and health centres), preventive services and family planning. A lot of the key raw material for the future planning of the service sits waiting to be mined from these cost statements.

The whole format of the annual accounts is currently being reviewed as part of the Körner review on Health Service information, and it is hoped that an improved set of standard accounts will emerge. There is certainly likely to be an emphasis on producing specialty costs as part of the minimum data set and encouragement for better methods of producing costs analysed by health care groups (the elderly, the mentally ill, etc.). It is also hoped that more experiments into ward and individual patient costing will be stimulated. There are a number of interesting local developments in producing innovative cost data and nurse managers should approach their treasurers to enquire what is available. Many treasurers are also producing imaginative annual financial reports for local consumption and nurse managers are encouraged to get hold of such reports.

Audit

Three types of audit operate within the NHS and they provide further key elements of the accountability mechanism:

1. Exchequer and audit – this is the Treasury's audit arm and the key method of probing central government expenditure and efficiency. They make periodic forays into the NHS.
2. DHSS audit – statutory external audit is normally provided by the DHSS Audit Branch (although the external audit for some Health Authorities has been put out to contract with firms of chartered accountants). The DHSS audit visit each Health Authority at least twice a year.
3. Internal audit – each Health Authority has an internal audit responsibility. Most Health Authorities employ their own auditors, but some Authorities have gone out to contract or have set up internal audit consortia on a multi-Authority basis.

The job of auditors is to review and report on:

- the adequacy of financial and other management controls;
- the extent of compliance with established policies, plans and procedures;
- the extent to which the organisation's assets are accounted for and safeguarded from losses of all kinds;
- the suitability and reliability of the organisation's management data.

Nurse managers should regard Internal Audit as an important resource to aid the management of their services and not as visitors from another planet who ask strange questions. Nurse managers should commission audit studies and use audit to probe how their organisation actually operates. Nurse managers should train auditors and vice versa.

Public accountability

The NHS is a public service and all managers must expect to be publicly accountable for their financial decisions (or the lack of them). In Parliament, the Select Committee on Social Services and the Public Accounts Committee scrutinise the NHS on a national basis. MPs can and do ask very specific questions on items of NHS expenditure. Ministers who are vulnerable to parliamentary criticism of their apparent lack of control feel obliged to set up ministerial review systems to probe the performance of Regions and to push Regions into holding Districts responsible to Regions in the same manner. District Health Authorities rightly probe the financial judgements of their senior officers and Community Health Councils seek financial information from the consumers' point of view.

THE FAMILY PRACTITIONER SERVICES

Nurse managers will be aware that family practitioners (doctors, dentists, chemists and ophthalmic practitioners and opticians) are independent contractors. A major dilemma for the NHS and the Treasury is that the expenditure generated by family practitioners is not subject to cash limits. The Government has unfortunately moved away from the loose integration of Family Practitioner Committees (FPCs) on the 1974 model and favours independent Health Authority status for FPCs. However, the search for a control mechanism continues and at national level, the expansion of the open-ended budget for family practitioner services clearly diminishes the resources that might have been available for the NHS as a whole. The decisions of family practitioners do have financial implications for nurse managers at local level. For example, expenditure on drugs and medical supplies in hospitals and community services is a charge on the finite Health Authority budgets. Similar expenditure generated by family practitioners is chargeable to the FPCs' open-ended budget. Over-prescribing by GPs can arouse patient expectation and lessen concern for the cost of resources.

Nurse managers will also be aware of a number of potential areas of possible overlap and duplication between GP and community health services, for example, vaccination and immunisation, family planning, screening and ante-natal care. The mode of provision of such services needs careful planning and evaluation to ensure comprehensive coverage, but to avoid overkill from multiple agencies. Fees per item of service are a significant part of GP remuneration and this can generate differences of interest between GPs and the salaried community health staff.

TRUST FUNDS AND FUND-RAISING

Trust Funds (also known as endowments or free monies) have accumulated over the years as a result of donations, legacies and the returns on investments of funds. It should be noted that Health Authorities have powers only to receive and administer donations in relation to health services.

The Trust Funds can be divided into three categories:

General Purpose
Special Purpose
Capital in Perpetuity (which may be General or Special)

It will be appreciated that the General Purpose Funds can be applied fairly broadly for health purposes. The Special Purpose Funds have to be applied more narrowly in accordance with the wishes of the donor. Capital in Perpetuity Funds are even more tightly prescribed as only the interest on the funds may be spent.

Trust Funds have traditionally been spent on research, amenities for staff and patients, and extra items of equipment which Exchequer funds have been unable to provide. The Health Authority has the duty of deciding what expenditure is appropriate, subject to any specific directions from the Secretary of State. For example, it is illegal to supplement the remuneration of staff from Trust Funds. It would also be inappropriate to use Trust Funds to meet the basic running costs of the service. However, in recent years expenditure from trust funds has become more varied and innovative and some quite substantial schemes have been funded (in whole or in part) from special donations.

The Trust Funds of Health Authorities have charitable status and the conduct of the Trust is governed by the law affecting Trustees. The principal advantage of this position is that the Trust Fund investments are exempt from income tax and capital gains tax, and a wide range of purchases from

Trust Funds are zero-rated for VAT. Also donations under a covenant for a period of more than three years to the Trust Funds of Authorities can qualify for repayment of tax.

The Authority and its officers have the normal duties of a trustee which include ensuring that money is spent in accordance with the objectives of the Trust and ensuring that proper accounts are kept.

Nurse managers should be actively involved in the management of Trust Funds at Unit level (Trust Funds are primarily a Unit resource although some Districts have central funds).

Until recently, Health Authorities have only had powers to receive, hold and administer Trust Funds. However, the 1980 Health Services Act gave Authorities the powers to actively engage in fund-raising. This can include the seeking of sponsorship, the launching of appeals and the running of fêtes and small lotteries. The powers have not been widely used by Health Authorities, particularly those who are already well served by Leagues of Friends and other voluntary agencies.

Clearly, there has been a desire to avoid fund-raising initiatives in competition with these groups, but successful appeals have been launched by Health Authorities for some projects. Nurse managers are ideal candidates to spearhead fund-raising activities. They also have a vital role in ensuring close cooperation between Health Authorities and voluntary agencies who raise funds for health projects in the District.

Fund-raising for particular pieces of equipment (especially diagnostic equipment) is now quite common. Nurse managers should use their influence to ensure proper value for money in such activity. Authorities also have to be cautious in accepting gifts of expensive equipment if there are significant revenue consequences which (unless they are also donated) can divert resources (including nursing staff) from current priorities.

FINANCIAL CONTROL – LOOKING AFTER OUR ASSETS

The treasurer has the job of accounting for movements in assets and liabilities. The balance sheet of a Health Authority is unusual in that it contains no capital assets or liabilities. However, it does contain current assets such as stock, debtors and cash and current liabilities (such as creditors) and the treasurer must ensure proper control of these balances throughout the organisation. In Health Authorities, much of the detailed financial control is delegated to general offices at Unit level, although nurse managers have an increasing role in this area.

The standing financial instructions

An essential part of financial control is the preparation and operation of standing financial instructions (SFIs). SFIs are issued by all Authorities in accordance with directions issued by the Secretary of State under the provision of the NHS Act 1977 for the regulation of the conduct of the Authority, its members and officers in relation to all financial matters.

The SFIs will cover a number of subjects including budgets, banking, security of assets, payments to staff and suppliers, contracting and purchasing, stores, income, patients' property, data processing, audit, condemning procedures, losses and trust funds. Many Authorities also produce detailed supplementary procedures for parts of the SFIs for relevant managers.

All nurse managers should have a copy of their Authority's SFIs and should be familiar with its contents. The SFIs should be sensible, intelligible and precise. If nurse managers have any difficulty in understanding them, they should tell their treasurer. Clearly, nurse managers have a major role to play in financial control systems. Indeed, all managers (and staff) have a general responsibility for the security of the assets of the Authority, for avoiding loss and for due economy in the use of resources.

Payment of salaries

Nursing officers should take their responsibility for pay nominations seriously and ensure that systems are properly designed and operated to ensure correct payments to staff. Failures in such systems will inevitably rebound on the nurse manager in terms of time-consuming case work, so it is well worth ensuring that they work properly, even if the routine procedures are completely delegated to nursing clerical staff.

The initial contract documentation is particularly vital in getting staff on to the payroll correctly and the same is true of documentation for termination. Nurse managers should ensure that there is proper certification of time sheets by designated officers, with due attention to sickness, overtime, unsocial hours, enhancements, etc. The flow of pay data from the employee through the nursing (or general office) to the treasurer's payroll department should be streamlined and yet secure against falsification of claims. Nurse managers should use the expertise in treasurers' departments to explain the requirements of these procedures to their staff (and their colleagues). Nurse managers also need to be properly acquainted with the Nursing Whitley Council's handbook on pay and conditions of service.

Payment of expenses

Similar principles apply to the payment of expenses to staff. Nurse managers should be familiar with the Whitley General Council handbook on matters like travelling expenses, removal expenses and excess rent. If in doubt, they should seek advice from the treasurer or local administrator before making any commitments. They should ensure that staff claims are properly checked and certified.

Supplies

Nurse managers should be well versed in the supplies systems that operate in their Authorities. These systems should be simple and effective and secure against fraud and misappropriation. There should be proper separation of duties with clear definitions of individual responsibilities. Nurse managers should probe the following questions:

Who is authorised to requisition?
Who has access to supplies held at ward level?
Who monitors consumption levels?
Do nurse managers have adequate influence in purchasing and contracting arrangements?
Is there an adequate flow of information on the quality and price of articles?
Are there sound condemning procedures for items such as patients' clothing, bedding and linen?

Income

Health Authorities have a number of statutory sources of income. The main ones are road traffic accident charges, private patients' income, charges to overseas visitors and charges for prescriptions and appliances. There are also a number of charges known as direct credits (these are mainly charges to staff such as meal charges, rent and lodging charges, laundry charges).

Both income and direct credits are retained locally by the Health Authority and help offset expenditure. Nurse managers will therefore appreciate that any evasion of charges or misappropriation of income will diminish the resources available locally for patient care. They should therefore offer any assistance needed by the treasurer or the local administrator to ensure both the correct recovery of income and the achievement of the maximum income yield (for example, schools of nursing need good information systems to ensure that staff accommodation is fully utilised and generates all the relevant income).

Stocks and inventories

Nurse managers will be aware that items held in stores are accounted for in terms of receipts, issues and balances held. It is thereby possible to charge budget managers for the consumption they generate by requisitioning supplies. As far as equipment is concerned, there are formidable problems in maintaining comprehensive inventories and the practice has tended to lapse, except in a few specialist areas. Many Authorities are now reviewing their policies in this area because of the need to plan investment in the context of proper knowledge of the present state of their assets and to tackle the problem of security of valuable equipment.

Nurse managers should give proper attention to the maintenance of inventories for relevant types of equipment under their control. Equipment to be considered is likely to be desirable, portable and valuable.

Losses and compensation

All managers have a responsibility for avoiding losses due to negligence, theft, fraud or arson and for reporting such losses to the local administrator and/or the treasurer. There is evidence that the formal records of losses maintained by treasurers considerably understate the real level of losses incurred by the NHS by waste or pilfering. Nurse managers have a particular responsibility to encourage responsibility and vigilance among their staff.

Compensation payments to staff or patients are another source of loss to an Authority's resources. There is a worrying trend towards more litigation and higher compensation awards. The nurse manager's skills are vital to the prevention of escalation in this area.

Nurse managers should be aware that Health Authorities carry no insurance cover (except for certain specialised equipment such as boilers where insurance is part of a maintenance contract) and therefore have to make good all losses from their budgets.

Patients' property

Health Authorities have a responsibility to provide safe custody for money and other personal property handed in by patients, or in the possession of unconscious, confused or dead patients. The treasurer provides written instruction on the collection, custody, recording, safekeeping and disposal of patients' property. Nurse managers should ensure that they and their staff are totally familiar with these procedures and that they know where their responsibilities lie. Mistakes and omissions can be both stressful and time-consuming.

FINANCIAL MANAGEMENT – ACHIEVING VALUE FOR MONEY

Nurse managers are in the front line of the struggle for better financial management in the NHS. The era of growth of financial resources has ended but the escalation of demand continues. There has never been a greater need to increase value for money in the organisation and delivery of services.

A financial squeeze has been applied in several directions. First, the top down squeeze stems from Government decisions not to fully fund pay awards or price inflation or to fund growth entirely from efficiency saving targets. Secondly, technological developments, medical and scientific advances generate pressures to provide more complex and expensive services to individual patients. Thirdly, the population's changing age structure and morbidity pattern is imposing pressures on volume and duration of service provision.

Nurse managers need to understand and influence the financial policies within which they operate. This should include an understanding of the overall District financial strategy.

Budgetary control

There is a small (but dwindling) band of nurse managers who are unenthusiastic about budgeting. They are heard to argue 'we used to "manage" without budgets', 'money is a problem for treasurers not nurse managers', 'we have to ensure the patient's welfare comes first', 'we only use what we need', 'we're no good at figures'. Anyone unlucky enough to encounter such a 'manager' could point out that budgeting is an aid to the manager's central tasks of planning, controlling and evaluating. Proper budgeting enables nurse managers to determine levels of service, to set standards and to agree priorities, to compare actual performance with expected performance. An effective budgetary system is one of the key methods of encouraging better use of resources as well as enabling Health Authorities to live within resource allocation. Budgeting should be a discipline but not a strait-jacket that will stifle initiative. It is a way of involving a wide range of managers in economic decisions. Budgeting is not just a financial exercise, it is a means of converting operational plans into action. Budgets should therefore contain manpower and workload measurements as well as costs. They are a means of quantifying an organisation's objectives and of pinpointing its weaknesses. The overall aim of budgeting is to reduce or maintain costs while maintaining or developing the quantity and quality of services.

Most budgeting systems in the NHS have been built on functional building blocks. In other words, budgets have been identified to match the responsibilities and work programmes of departmental managers. This does not rule out the possibility of building budget information in other dimensions and work is being undertaken to analyse expenditure by medical and surgical specialty as a base for planning future expenditure and as a means of reaching understanding with clinicians on resource use.

Defining the budget content

The content of each budget should be defined to reflect the source of decision-making on commitment and expenditure (for example, signing requisitions, hiring staff). The classification of expenditure headings must be defined and agreed with all managers to encompass all types of expenditure. The budget should also contain a defined manpower plan for the year in terms of numbers and grades of staff. Manpower plans must be based on planned rotas with an appropriate definition of levels of enhancement, overtime or on-call provision. This manpower plan must be drawn up as part of the budget setting exercise. Budgets should also be set to reflect defined activity levels and service objectives.

The analysis of income and expenditure

Effective budgetary management requires an expenditure analysis which is reliable and pitched to the right level of detail. This necessitates an effective system of coding, incorporating validation checks but largely carried out at budget manager level or below. The coding structure will normally define expenditure subjectively by department and by location. Some budgets may incorporate a specialty or care group dimension. The accounts system should be able to consolidate this coding information in several dimensions with appropriate summaries or extracts to meet the needs of managers. Nurse managers should think through their needs for expenditure analysis and assist in designing coding structures and report formats.

Defining the powers of budget managers

A budget manager is responsible for managing his service within his budget which should be designed to cover the basic ongoing costs of his department, taking into account the defined level of service. He should be given maximum flexibility to switch money between expenditure heads within defined parameters.

To encourage savings and better use of resources, budget managers must be able to influence the way those savings are used. Districts should define financial limits (which may vary between recurring and non-recurring savings) for decision by budget managers on redeployment.

Maximum flexibility on virement (transfers between budget headings) is also desirable, providing that virement is consistent with budget objectives. Policies on virement and use of savings usually contain check lists on points to be satisfied before virement goes ahead, such as:

- Will appropriate standards of care of service be maintained?
- Are budget changes consistent with planning objectives?
- Have the proposals been properly evaluated?
- In particular, will non-recurring expenditure from savings generate extra recurring costs?

The minimum data set for budgetary control

Detailed requirements will vary between managers and between functions but reporting systems should be designed to ensure all relevant detail is provided at budget manager level with appropriate summary reports for senior managers, Unit teams, the DMT and the Authority.

In order to exercise proper control, budget managers should give attention on a regular basis to:

1. Budgeted and actual levels of activity.
2. The annual budget analysed by staff grade and type of non-staff expenditure.
3. The budget and expenditure (or income) for the month, with suitable analysis.
4. The budget and expenditure (or income) for the period to date with suitable analysis (including commitments where relevant).
5. Variance analysis of over- and under-spending for the period to date.
6. The budgeted and actual staffing level by grade and whole-time equivalent. Staff can be grouped by pay scale to indicate skill mix.

7. *Ad hoc* additional information on problem areas (for example, level of staff absence and turnover).

On the question of manpower control, the Körner Manpower Working Party has offered a useful definition which encompasses the following:

- limiting employment to a predetermined budget level,
- efficient use, the way in which staff are used, for example, the control of rotas, overtime and absences,
- effective use, for example, the balance of trained and untrained staff, staff development and the combining of various staff skills and grades to obtain the optimum combination of volume and quality of throughput at allowed budget cost.

Budget reporting systems

Regular financial statements should provide information to nurse managers on such items as:

1. Budget and expected level of activity.
2. The proportion of budget to end of current period; monthly budget.
3. Expenditure/income to the end of the period; expenditure/income for the last month (this may make the identification of trends easier).
4. Variance to date and (if useful) projected variances to the end of the financial year, and commitments incurred.
5. Manpower – planned staffing levels,
   – actual in post,
   – moving average in post for current period.
6. Additional information for specific problem areas and appropriate exception reports.

Table 3 is an illustration of a typical budget statement for a nurse manager.

The role of the management accountant

The role of the management accountant is to act as financial adviser to the budget manager. In this task the principal aspects are the preparation of annual budgets and supporting documentation and the updating of budgets at pay and price increases, etc. The management accountant also produces

05 Months to month 05 (rounded – units of £1)	Line No.	MPE this month Budget	MPE this month Actual	Nursing Staff Services – Hospital No. Annual budget £	Report Set No. 100 This month Budget £	This month Expend. £	Report Number Form No. 400 Loc. No. 119 Budget for period £	Column Layout d Expend. for period £	Over/ under(–) £
Salaries and Wages									
Nursing Officer	04	1.00	1.00	9,605	801	784	4,005	4,129	124
Sisters/Charge Nurses	14	5.78	5.00	49,940	4,162	3,666	20,810	18,704	2,106–
Community Sisters/Charge Nurses	16								
Staff Nurses	19	7.34	6.56	47,644	3,971	3,685	19,855	19,424	431–
Senior SENs	24	1.49	0.85	10,068	839	501	4,195	2,579	1,616–
SENs	25	10.09	9.93	59,612	4,967	5,226	24,835	26,231	1,396
Nursing Aux/Assts	27	37.44	30.38	182,895	15,241	12,554	76,205	67,653	8,552–
Bank Nurses – SRN	30		1.57			1,334		5,628	5,628
Bank Nurses – SEN	31		0.55			341		1,786	1,786
Students	33								
Pupils	35								
Agency Nurses – Trained	37					652		730	730
Agency Nurses – Untrained	38					694		954	954
Total Salaries and Wages	60	63.14	55.84	359,764	29,981	29,438	149,905	147,817	2,088–
Other Expenditure									
Dressings	61			6,504	548	530	2,678	2,437	241–
CSSD packs	62								
M & S supplies – disposable	72			6,161	517	263	2,538	1,249	1,289–
Surgical instruments	78								
Staff uniforms	81								
Surgical gloves	82			498	41	35	205	168	37–
Patients' clothing	84			2,878	241	257	1,197	1,274	77
Bedding and linen – disposables	85			1,626	136	894	680	3,885	3,205
B & L – sheepskin items	86			25	2		10		10–
Travel and subsistence	93								
Total Other Expenditure	98			17,692	1,485	1,978	7,308	9,013	1,705
Total – Gross Expenditure	99	63.14	55.84	377,456	31,466	31,416	157,213	156,830	383–

Reproduced with kind permission of the East Dorset Health Authority.

monthly statements of performance against budget and comments on variances. He should assist the budget manager in monitoring expenditure trends and obtaining better value for money through *ad hoc* cost investigations.

Conclusion

Each District should have a written budgetary procedure document with explicit definitions of the issues outlined above. Nurse managers who do not possess such a document should approach their treasurers. Better still, nurse managers should be involved in writing such documents. Nurse managers should not be content with managing their own budgets; they should understand and influence the District's budgetary strategy on issues like development funds (or the lack of them), non-recurring programmes, holding of reserves (general or specific).

Financial planning

The financial information which is required for operational planning (two to three years ahead) and for budgeting (one year ahead) is similar in kind to that required for strategic planning (up to ten years ahead). The information for operational planning must normally be more detailed and more precise than that for strategic planning. Managers and planners need information on:

Resources. The capital and revenue resources currently available and the planned allocations of resources (that is, resource assumption) for future years. Planning has normally been conducted in volume (constant price) terms but there is inevitably some uncertainty about future allocations and the uncertainty has increased substantially with the introduction of cash planning. This means that future resource assumptions may be varied by the over- or under-funding of inflation.

The cost of existing services. Expenditure on particular services should be related to the most appropriate units of activity. Districts can analyse their costs as fixed, semi-variable and variable, and thus calculate the variable costs of their activities. Also, different types of expenditure vary according to different criteria, for example, length of patient stay, volume of patient throughput, volume of buildings, etc. From this information managers and planners can develop estimates of costs for different levels of activities and assess trends in costs. In this context marginal costs may have much more significance than average costs (marginal cost is the extra cost incurred, or saved, by a change in the volume of an activity).

The range of options for the development and maintenance of services. This may include the cost of improving services for a particular care group, or the revenue consequences of individual capital schemes, or the potential cost/savings related to changes in operational plan. The timing as well as the magnitude of the costs may be important.

Investment appraisal. Before capital resources are spent, the Authority should be satisfied that any development is justified in terms of its priorities and that it is an appropriate size and design. The appraisal should include a clear exposition of costs and benefits and the appraisal of cash flow generated by the project.

Sensitivity of factors to change. Financial planning must take into account the sensitivity of the various elements of the appraisal to changes in the component data. For example, the viability of some projects may be affected by a relatively small shift in the estimates of costs or benefits.

It is hoped that nurse managers will play a much greater role at Unit, District and Region in the formulation and evaluation of planning proposals. They should not overlook opportunities provided by joint planning and joint financing to put forward more innovative proposals for community-based health care. They should also not shrink from the rigorous re-planning of currently provided services. Planning is basically about reviewing the value of existing services, not about preparing shopping lists of desirable extras.

Evaluation and performance review

Nurse managers will also need financial information to help evaluate the efficiency with which services are provided. Cost information in this context should help probe performance standards and the value for money of current services; better information should lead to better judgements on both effectiveness and efficiency. It may involve comparisons between services and different Units/Districts or between similar methods of meeting similar service requirements, or between similar services over periods of time. Costing for performance review tends to be in depth and more *ad hoc* than that required for planning and budgeting, but the activity of performance review should be a routine one. It is clearly important that results of performance reviews should be fed back to improve the quality of future budgets and plans.

MANAGEMENT COSTS

The Secretary of State has stated that restraint of management costs must continue and that by 1984/85 each Region will be required to achieve a level of management costs 10 per cent below the national level obtained in 1979/80. This saving is seen to be one of the principal objectives of the 1982 reorganisation. The national management costs figure for 1979/80, expressed as a percentage of national turnover, was announced at 5.13 per cent. Therefore, by 1984/85, the management cost percentage for each Region will need to be no greater than 4.62 per cent of Regional turnover (turnover is broadly defined as capital and revenue expenditure plus income).

Regions in turn have to set management cost targets for their own headquarters and their District Health Authorities consistent with the overall objective. Districts in turn have had to be careful to plan their revised structures, both within their management costs targets and within what they can afford in real cash terms.

Management costs have been defined by the DHSS in considerable detail in terms of accounting classifications. In summary, the following types of expenditure are defined as management costs within a District:

- All administrative and clerical staff employed on District Headquarters functions (including FPC) and all staff employed at Unit level graded Senior Administrative Assistant and above.
- District Medical Officer and District Dental Officer (the latter is spending more than 50 per cent of his time on administration).
- Nursing staff graded Director of Nursing Services and above, Senior Nurses (staff support) and Senior Nurses who have other Senior Nurses reporting to them.
- Any headquarters-based Pharmaceutical Officers.
- District Advisers (and the Senior Manager for each function if he has District-wide responsibilities) for Catering, Domestic, CSSD and Laundry Services.
- Ambulance Officers in Grades 1 to 4.
- District Works Officers and Senior Support staff.
- Chairman's remuneration and members' expenses.
- In addition, 100 per cent of headquarters non-staff costs are included.

There is a clear government commitment to the continuation of management costs control despite the low percentage of management costs in the NHS in relation to national and international comparisons. This control may inhibit investment in better management of the service by imposing criteria other than normal measurement of costs and benefits. It may also stimulate managers to design and operate within simple and streamlined management structures. Nurse managers can take a lead here, both within their own discipline and by constructive criticism of the management structures of other disciplines. Management structures set up on 1982 should be regularly reappraised to check on their continuing effectiveness and not left to atrophy for all time.

THE DEVELOPMENT OF FINANCIAL INFORMATION SYSTEMS

There are three major national standard systems in widespread use for financial purposes:

1. Standard Payroll System (SPS) – this is a highly standard system. SPS (or its equivalent in regions not using SPS) is both a payment system and a major data base for Health Service management.
2. The Standard Manpower Planning Information System (STAMP) – this feeds off SPS and has standard modules as well as facilities to design *ad hoc* reports.
3. Standard Accounting System (SAS) – this is, in fact, a non-standard system in accounting terms, as there is local flexibility in designing coding structures and reporting formats. However, the basic system is designed to achieve the two key objectives of any accounting system: the maintenance of financial control by accounting for all transactions and the provision of financial information, by analysing those transactions into a wide range of classifications.

Regions which do not use the national standard systems have developed (or borrowed) alternatives which meet similar objectives.

Hitherto, most computer systems have tended to be orientated to individual applications with interfaces with other systems where appropriate, for example, supplies and stock control systems linked with stores accounting systems, payroll systems and creditor payments feeding into the accounting systems.

Nurse managers at all levels will hopefully already be involved in the development of information systems. The trend is clearly towards systems that link patient activity, manpower and financial data. All systems need to be related to a comprehensive District information strategy.

Nurse managers should be aware of the trend towards a local design of information systems for minicomputers and microcomputers and be prepared to participate in their design.

FINANCIAL TRAINING FOR NURSE MANAGERS

Nurse managers carry a responsibility for training themselves and their subordinates in financial management. Indeed, nurse managers with a good grasp of financial management can play a major role in the training of other managers and clinicians because of their added perspective as nurse managers.

Nurse managers should develop a good working relationship with the treasurer and his senior staff. They have a lot to learn from each other. Treasurers can contribute to nurse training at student and post-basic levels. Treasurers also need training to appreciate the problems of the nurse manager.

THE NURSE MANAGER AND THE TREASURER

An effective working relationship between nurse managers and the treasurer's department can exert a major influence over the management style of the Authority. Jointly, they can make a major contribution to the effective management and development of the Authority's services.

Nurse managers have the right to expect the treasurer to provide an effective and comprehensive paymaster service. Their constructive criticism will be welcomed, but they must be willing to play their part in the paymaster system, for example, in ensuring that pay nominations are properly made, that expense claims are properly certified, that requisitions and ordering procedures are adhered to.

An active interest by nurse managers in management information can stimulate the treasurer to improve his information performance. This should be an interactive process as there is no value in the treasurer producing information that the nurse manager cannot use or understand.

CONCLUSION

The management of health service finance presents many complex and challenging problems but, contrary to the belief of some treasurers and many nurse managers, it need not be a mysterious and obscure process. Indeed, a good grasp of health service finances should be quite within the scope of any self-respecting nurse manager.

Suggested further reading

Association of Health Service Treasurers: *Patients' Property, Income and Allowances.*
Association of Health Service Treasurers: *Non-exchequer Funds.*
Association of Health Service Treasurers: *The Role of the Treasurer.*
Association of Health Service Treasurers: *Internal Audit in the NHS.*
East Dorset Health Authority (annual publication) *Budgetary Policy and Guidelines for Managers.*
Institute of Health Service Administrators: *Health Care in the United Kingdom – Its Organisation and Management.*
Jones, T. & Prowle, M. *Health Service Finance: An Introduction.* London: Certified Accountants Educational Trust.
King Edward's Hospital Fund for London: *Accounting for Health.*
Report of the Financial Working Party of the Steering Group on Health Services Information (the Körner Committee).
Royal Commission Research Paper No. 2 (The Perrin Report) *The Management of Financial Resources in the National Health Service.*

Chapter 8
Managing Education

JANICE CACKETT

The next five years are a time of challenge and opportunity for nurse education. The new statutory bodies, the National Boards and the United Kingdom Central Council for Nursing, Midwifery and Health Visiting, became operational in July 1983. Future educational policies have yet to be decided. The issues being discussed include the future preparation for nursing, the level of qualifications, the pattern of continuing education and recurrent registration on evidence of continuing education. Recognition of the need for change and for continuing professional education provides the managers of nurse education with scope for exciting initiatives. This chapter discusses the management of nurse education within the National Health Service from three perspectives: first, the management of nurse education programmes at basic and post-basic level; secondly, the management of the school of nursing; and thirdly, the management of education within the nursing management structure. Initially, education and management are briefly defined and their interrelationship discussed.

Education is a concept with numerous definitions, but essentially it is concerned with developing the potential of each individual and with facilitating this. Stenhouse (1975) identifies four components of education: training, instruction, initiation and induction. Training is concerned with the acquisition of skills, the correct performance of which requires practice under supervision; instruction is concerned with teaching/learning with direct information-giving (the cognitive aspects of the learning process), initiation with the absorption of the values and attitude of the institution, often intangible, and induction is concerned with higher-level thinking, the development of conceptual skills, broad principles and individual potential. Nursing education, through a variety of activities at basic and post-basic level, encompasses each of these areas, some of which will be discussed in this chapter.

Management theory has evolved in the last 80 years. The different schools of management theory, for example, scientific management, human relations school, and classical management, have been referred to earlier. In this chapter, the term 'management' is used to include planning, organising, leading and controlling the activities being undertaken by people within an organisation.

Planning is concerned with forecasting need, deciding and stating aims to be achieved and suggesting the method to attain these, taking account of organisational constraints and resources. Organising involves using resources, people and time effectively to attain the aims of the organisation, ensuring that individuals have the knowledge and skills to fulfil their role. Leading involves directing and motivating the human resources within an organisation, controlling and monitoring the effectiveness of the individual within the organisation and the work of the total institution against agreed standards of performance. It is the blending of these two concepts of management and education that provides the challenge in the management of nurse education within the health system. First, the management of basic and post-basic nurse education programmes is discussed.

THE MANAGEMENT OF BASIC AND POST-BASIC NURSE EDUCATION PROGRAMMES

Basic programmes

Basic programmes are programmes that lead to an initial statutory qualification. The recognised statutory qualifications in the United Kingdom are included in different parts of the professional register. They are as follows:

Part 1	Registered General Nurse	RGN
2	Enrolled Nurse (General)	EN(G)
3	Registered Mental Nurse	RMN
4	Enrolled Nurse (Mental)	EN(M)
5	Registered Nurse for the Mentally Handicapped	RNMH
6	Enrolled Nurse (Mental Handicap)	EN(MH)
7	Enrolled Nurse	EN
8	Registered Sick Children's Nurse	RSCN

The management of basic nurse education programmes is concerned with forecasting the needs of patients, the skills and knowledge required to meet these, and the number of nurses for the future. It includes providing the learning experience to equip individuals for practice in the immediate future and to instil an attitude that motivates them to continue to undertake learning activities to provide the knowledge base for future professional practice. The planning and organisation of basic nurse education is concerned with the learners, their learning experience and the sequence of this. It takes into account organisational constraints and resources.

Planning the basic programme requires all involved to discuss and decide the aims of the programmes. In the United Kingdom, the recently published Statutory Instrument states the expected competency level on completion of the programme leading to the different parts of the professional register:

Training for admission to Parts 1 – 8 of the Register

1. Courses leading to a qualification, the successful completion of which shall enable an application to be made for admission to Part 1, 3, 5 or 8 of the Register, shall provide opportunities to enable the student to accept responsibility for her professional development and to acquire the competencies required to:

   (a) advise on the promotion of health and the prevention of illness
   (b) recognise situations that may be detrimental to the health and well-being of the individual
   (c) carry out activities involved when conducting the comprehensive assessment of a person's nursing requirements
   (d) recognise the significance of the observations made and use these to develop an initial nursing assessment
   (e) devise a plan of nursing care based on the assessment with the cooperation of the patient, to the extent that this is possible, taking into account the medical prescription
   (f) implement the planned programme of nursing care and where appropriate teach and coordinate other members of the caring team who may be responsible for implementing specific aspects of the nursing care
   (g) review the effectiveness of the nursing care provided and where appropriate, initiate any action that may be required
   (h) work in a team with other nurses, and with medical and paramedical staff and social workers
   (i) undertake the management of the care of a group of patients over a period of time and organise the appropriate support services

   related to the care of the particular type of patient with whom she is likely to come in contact when registered in that Part of the Register for which the student intends to qualify.

2. Courses leading to a qualification, the successful completion of which shall enable an application to be made for admission to Part 2, 4, 6 or 7 of the Register, shall be designed to prepare the student to undertake

nursing care under the direction of a person registered in Part 1, 3, 5 or 8 of the Register and provide opportunities for the student to develop the competencies required to:

(a) assist in carrying out comprehensive observation of the patient and help in assessing her care requirements
(b) develop skills to enable her to assist in the implementation of nursing care under the direction of a person registered in Part 1, 3, 5 or 8 of the Register
(c) accept delegated nursing tasks
(d) assist in reviewing the effectiveness of the care provided
(e) work in a team with other nurses, and with medical and paramedical staff and social workers

related to the care of the particular type of patient with whom she is likely to come into contact when registered in that Part of the Register for which the student intends to qualify.

(Statutory Instrument 1983, No. 873, pp. 10 to 11)

The above provides a broad statement of the aims of the programme and thus the parameters within which to develop curriculum plans. Detailed curriculum planning considers the aims of the programme, the learning activities, their assessment and evaluation; the curriculum has to be meaningful and relevant to the learners, and is a dynamic concept changing in response to continual evaluation.

There are many definitions of 'curriculum'. Kerr (1968) defined it in this way: 'The curriculum is all the learning which is planned and guided by the School whether it is carried on in groups or individually, inside or outside the School.' 'Curriculum' encompasses the totality of the learning experiences and those involved in them. It includes both the overt learning experience and the covert learning which absorbs the culture of the organisation – the induction discussed by Stenhouse and included in the 'hidden curriculum' of most curriculum theorists.

Factors influencing curriculum development in nursing are illustrated in Figure 3. Curriculum planning and development is usually undertaken by a group representing all parts of the training circuit including nurse teachers, nurse managers, clinical nurses and nurse learners. The group discusses all aspects of the curriculum, receives information about its effectiveness and makes recommendations for change.

Guidance in curriculum planning for basic nurse education is provided in the education policy document 77/19 and the updated statement 83/13 from the previous Statutory Body, the General Nursing Council for England and

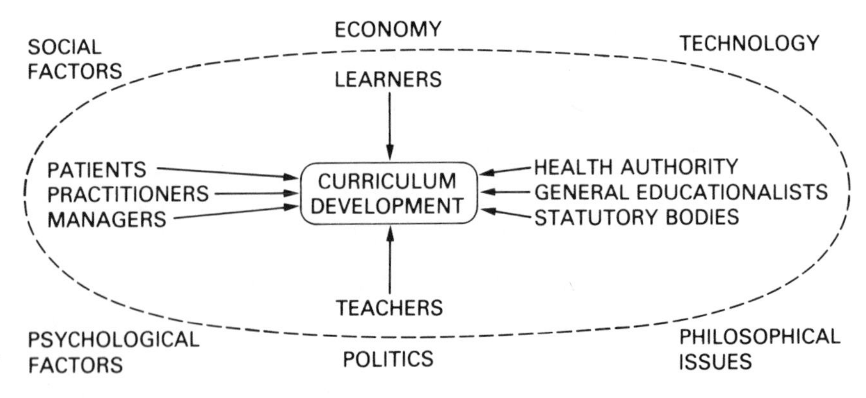

Figure 3. Factors influencing curriculum development.

Wales. Many of the issues discussed in this section are included in their documents.

Selection of learners

The management of the selection of learners should ideally include decisions on the numbers required to enter nursing in order to meet future demands. However, bearing in mind that the basic programmes are, at present, the way of entry into all post-basic training programmes and opportunities, this task involves careful manpower planning. Factors to consider in deciding numbers are the availability of teachers, the clinical experience, the availability of trained staff supervision, the financial consequences and, particularly where mobility is limited, the employment prospects on qualification.

Once the numbers are decided, management of the selection process is concerned with deciding criteria for selection and how these might be tested. Criteria for selection have to be agreed by all involved in teaching and supporting the learners and usually include academic criteria and personal qualities. Academic criteria are objective, easily identified and can be checked; personal qualities are subjective and difficult to assess. Academic criteria are usually defined by the Statutory Body and from July 1986 will, in the United Kingdom, be five 'O' levels or the equivalent; personal qualities usually include evidence of working with people and in a team, ability to communicate and a high level of motivation and insight into the demands of the role. The actual selection process should provide the candidate with the opportunity to assess the environment within which she may work, thus emphasising the partnership between the learner, the school and the environment where learning occurs. Interviews are conducted by two people, one from the clinical area and one from the school. Criteria usually considered by prospective learners include the range of programmes available, the size and geographical location of the school and the facilities and atmosphere of the organisation.

The interview is planned so each knows the areas they will cover. The candidate should be informed of the result as soon as possible. At present, in England, because of the vast numbers applying to several schools of nursing, the idea of a central clearing house system for nurses is being considered. To this end, a common application form is now in widespread use and a common medical health screening form is being discussed.

Selection of learning experience

Having selected the learner, the management of basic nurse education aims to provide a dynamic curriculum which takes account of local facilities and the statutory requirements, both those of the national body and, if appropriate, of the European Economic Community. The overall requirement in terms of total hours for a training programme is stated. However, the length of time in each experience and the ordering of these is usually left to local decision and is approved by the Statutory Body. The clinical experiences have to meet specific criteria jointly agreed by ward and school staff. Research studies (Fretwell, 1980; Ogier, 1981 and Orton, 1981) have indicated criteria which meet the learning needs and provide a climate for learning; the circulars referred to above also suggest possible criteria. It is essential that these are used as a basis for local agreement. The criteria for learning wards may include the ratio of trained to untrained staff; evidence of planned individualised care; a ward sister/charge nurse with teaching qualifications or at least one demonstrating an interest in teaching and an awareness of learning needs. The sister/charge nurse should also be an assessor and show evidence of continuing professional development. Controlling the learning environment requires a team of teachers and service colleagues to monitor that all clinical areas meet the agreed criteria and to take appropriate action if this is not so; it is suggested such monitoring occurs on a twice-yearly basis.

Liaison with the school should be through a specific member of the teaching staff who participates in the clinical teaching and supervision of learners. The ward sister and the teacher can together identify the specific learning opportunities available during each experience and the expected outcome for each level of learning. The school is dependent on the commitment of trained staff in the clinical areas to provide supervision and to identify with each learner specific opportunities for learning. To achieve this, trained staff have to be involved in curriculum discussions, to know the content of the theoretical instruction and to be aware of the sequential pattern of the training programme. This knowledge should equip trained staff to understand, identify and agree the individual learner needs and assist their progress through training.

Sequential pattern of the training programme

The specific clinical experience must, as already discussed, meet the statutory requirements. The sequence of experience is decided locally and approved centrally.

The majority of programmes in England are at present based on the modular system or a modification of it. This pattern attempts to relate theory to practice by providing a period of preparation in the school, the relevant clinical experience and a period of consolidation. The sequence of the programme endeavours to ensure an even flow of learners to the clinical area, which is particularly vital in most parts of the United Kingdom where learners are employees of the Health Authority and thus contribute, in varying degrees, to the ward staff. Sequencing may also be related to the particular model of curriculum development, for example, if the basis is the biographical model it may start with maternity and child care. There is considerable variation in the sequence and trained staff should be aware of this in order to understand the level of knowledge and skill each learner brings to their area. Trained staff are expected to assess the clinical competence of learners; this assessment may be episodic or continuous.

The assessment of learners

The assessment of progress of learners includes assessment of their knowledge and of skills. Assessment of knowledge is usually through a series of formal written examinations and multiple-choice questions combined with project work, case histories and short-answer questions. Assessment takes place at agreed points throughout training and an examination has to be passed on completion of training for registration with the Statutory Body.

Assessment of clinical skills may be episodic or continuous. Episodic assessment occurs at specific points during training and includes the assessment of a particular aspect of care. The number and type of assessment is laid down for each type of statutory training. Learners' progress is also assessed by reports written by the trained staff for each area of clinical experience. In some schools, schemes of continuous assessment are implemented, following approval by the Statutory Body. Continuous practical assessment endeavours to assess the learner's progress throughout training and replaces both the episodic assessment and ward reports. Progress is related to the individual's development and acquisition of skills with summative points for each year of training. The trained staff, teaching staff and learners themselves contribute to this assessment.

The management of the assessment programme should ensure that all involved are aware of the assessment format and timetable. Learners and trained staff are given a clear indication of what is expected and guidelines for undertaking assessments. Planning assessments involves preparing trained staff for that role by assessors' workshops or study days, with an interview and discussion prior to appointment as an assessor. Observation of others undertaking assessments may be helpful. Clearly agreed criteria by which to measure progress of learners need to be established.

Monitoring assessment is by careful recording of the assessments undertaken by each learner and their results, and of the number undertaken by each assessor and their results. The continuous assessment scheme is reviewed by the teaching team at agreed points. Discussion of aspects of assessment and work of assessors at regular assessors' meetings also provides the opportunity for monitoring the scheme and discussing issues. Additionally, a small group meeting quarterly to discuss assessment referrals and failures adds to the monitoring system. As the vast majority of learners are full-time employees, a clear indication of the stage at which referral in assessment may ultimately result in discontinuation of training is essential.

The management of nurse education is not solely concerned with the programme leading to statutory qualifications but also with post-basic education activities.

Post-basic education

The term 'post-basic education' is used to include all aspects of staff development. It encompasses in-service training, continuing education, advanced clinical courses and staff development. Each of these areas is included in the framework of staff development and it is suggested that for these to be managed effectively, nurse managers and nurse teachers must collaborate closely.

It is essential for managers and educators to work together to ensure that those employed within the organisation are able to fulfil their role and their potential. It is suggested that for this to occur plans have to be made to ensure all staff are:

1. Prepared for the role and responsibilities they are expected to undertake.
2. Given opportunities to develop the skills and knowledge for their role and to use these effectively.
3. Given opportunities for annual 'updating', 'refreshing' in particular areas, for example, fire training, lifting techniques.
4. Professionally up-to-date.
5. Developed laterally by examining particular facets of their role.
6. Prepared for career progression.
7. Monitored against agreed performance standards.

It is noted that by 1990 all nurses will require evidence of continuing education in the previous five years to be eligible to practise.

In-service training

In-service training involves providing opportunities to enable staff to master the skills of their job, to learn new skills as their responsibility widens and to participate in annual updating programmes. In-service training should be provided for the complete range of nursing staff.

Initially, in-service training will ensure that all newly employed staff have an orientation programme to introduce them to the organisation, the people within it and the expectation of their role. It is vital to ensure that staff are trained for new techniques; the training for nurses to administer intravenous drugs is an example of how in-service training is provided to meet the extended role of the nurse. Specific in-service training may be identified at job and performance review with a senior nurse manager; needs for continuing education and staff development may also be identified during this process.

Advanced clinical courses

Continuing clinical education evolved under the auspices of the Joint Board of Clinical Nursing Studies and the mechanism for obtaining approval serves as an example of managing this aspect of post-basic education. The need for the course is identified in relation to the experience available, the availability of educational support, the geographical location and the level of financial support. 'Experience' includes the actual clinical experience, the level of trained, experienced staff for supervision and the demands of other learners on that experience. 'Educational support' includes qualified teachers, secretarial support and library resources being available. 'Geographical location' examines the feasibility of mounting a course within a Regional Health Authority. 'Financial support' has to consider the salaries of the course members, the support staff and costs of overheads.

The decision to run a course having been made, a planning team is convened to undertake the detailed planning of the course. Alongside the work of the planning team, preparation of those in the clinical areas for the teaching and assessing of post-basic students is necessary. Recruitment of students for a course with agreed criteria for selection should then ensure that an effective course is organised.

Continuing education and staff development

Continuing education for staff is the responsibility of the trained professional nurse and the employing Authority. Staff should be encouraged to read professional journals and library facilities should be available to them. Educational experience to enhance their performance could include such items as preparation for the role of a qualified nurse, development of teaching and assessing skills, report writing and development of counselling skills. The sequence, learning, and content of these courses, often arranged locally, require agreement and commitment from both managers and teachers.

The new Diploma in Nursing (London University), Diploma in Professional Studies (CNAA) and post-registration degree courses in nursing offer continuing education opportunities for qualified staff. The Diploma in Nursing is presently organised jointly between a school of nursing and an educational institution. The management of such a programme includes identifying the need, planning and organising the pattern, content and assessment and providing teaching input; resources for such a venture must be identified. Liaison with further and higher education is an important element in the management of continuing education. It should ensure the most effective use of skills and resources.

To assist in the effective use of resources, a policy for study leave for staff has to be discussed and agreed by the nursing policy-making group. The managers of both education and nursing services decide the number to be seconded to the course, criteria for selection and agreed selection procedures, degree of financial support and means for measuring the benefit of the educational experiences. The budget for study leave from the Health Authority may be held by the educational manager or service staff. In either case, a mechanism for disseminating information relating to opportunities for study leave, a method of screening these, identifying appropriate courses, the secondment procedure, briefing, debriefing and reporting has to be agreed. The agreed policy is then made available to all staff and reviewed annually.

Courses following registration leading to additional qualification include Midwifery, Health Visiting and District Nursing.

Midwifery education is in a state of change as the 18-month training has recently been introduced. Discussion continues concerning the relationships between the midwifery school and the school of nursing. Close relationships are vital to ensure peer group support, the sharing of educational ideas and economic use of resources. At the time of writing, the future organisational framework for midwifery education is not yet decided. The management of the basic training follows similar principles to those outlined above under 'Basic Programmes' and midwives have similar needs for staff development programmes. Additionally, the statutory requirement for five-yearly refresher courses has to be included in plans both in relation to replacement staff and costs.

Health visiting education is firmly established in further and higher education and district nurse education is just establishing its courses in the education sector. The educational manager in the National Health Service may be involved in such courses by participating in the selection for secondment to the course and by liaison with departments offering such courses in order to share experiences, ideas and professional knowledge.

THE MANAGEMENT OF A SCHOOL OF NURSING

Management of education in the Health Service is also concerned with the management of the educational organisation, the school of nursing. The newly created Statutory Bodies have yet to decide the overall management structure for schools of nursing. The present system is described below with the anticipation that much information will be transferable to any new system to be implemented.

Managing a school involves managing the staff, the teachers and support staff, the educational programme (discussed in the section above), financial management and evaluation; it is concerned with day-to-day administration, with planning, organising, leading and controlling the educational activities of the organisation and the staff within it.

The teaching staff

Management of the teachers includes selection, secondment, role function, development and monitoring of their performance. Teachers are experienced clinical nurses who have undertaken a further course of study to obtain a teaching qualification. They are a group of senior professional colleagues, each with particular skills to contribute to the whole. When managing the staff, their level of skill and achievement must be recognised.

The staffing structure may be on a team or specialist basis or a combination of these. It includes an agreed ratio of clinical teachers and tutors, senior tutors and occasionally, dependent on school size, an Assistant Director of Nurse Education.

The staff may be arranged in teams headed by a Senior Tutor with responsibility either for a particular level or area of teaching or for a particular group of learners. The arrangement should ensure that learners have personal support throughout training and teachers are able to use their specialist knowledge. The structure requires flexibility to ensure that this is achieved.

The selection of staff commences with secondment to a nurse teacher's course. In England this is available on full salary and with fees and expenses paid from central funds on the recommendation of the Director of Nurse Education who has agreed with service managers that the individual is clinically competent to teach.

Numerous courses are available. It is inappropriate to list them, but the potential teacher should consider geographical location and the qualification obtained as well as the content of the course. (Details are available in ENB Circular 8301). Selection of staff takes account of who has been seconded, the funded establishment and the particular skills required by the school. The number of tutorial staff for basic courses is determined by student numbers and they are presently funded separately from other tutorial staff. The particular role of the teacher in each school will vary according to the extent of team teaching, specialist teaching and clinical involvement; potential staff must clearly understand their role. Orientation of staff to the school and the ward areas is essential.

Leading the staff involves discussing, deciding and stating the aims of the school, the philosophy of nursing to which it is committed and the mechanism for achieving these. It includes deciding the structure of the school and the role of each teacher within it, motivating staff, encouraging educational innovation in a supportive environment and facilitating development and growth, ensuring both professional autonomy for the teacher and monitoring by the manager. An open system of communication is essential if this is to be achieved. Communication within the school should include information meetings, planning meetings and peer group discussion where teaching methods and experience can be shared. Such an environment should ensure support for newly qualified staff and opportunities for continued development of experienced staff.

Controlling staff includes monitoring the performance of teachers initially after six months then annually through a job and performance review. This provides the opportunity to assess the level of performance and the allocation of time, to identify training needs, discuss future career development and identify key tasks for the following year. Alongside this formal monitoring there is much informal monitoring resulting from team teaching, learner feedback and peer review. A work diary for a period of time may assist in assessing allocation of time and provide the basis for review discussion.

Training needs may include such areas as counselling skills, budgeting and industrial relations. Opportunities for undertaking courses in these areas may be provided with careful briefing and debriefing. Many teachers are encouraged to undertake part-time degree studies as the move towards a graduate profession is discussed. Secondment to courses where considerable time may be involved needs to be discussed and agreed by all members of the teaching team to ensure the workload is fairly distributed.

The non-teaching staff

Administrative support and the assistance of a librarian and audio-visual aids technician is vital to the efficient management of a school. Each should be able to clearly identify his contribution to the whole and his relationship with the teaching staff.

Secretarial staff are often led by a General Administrator responsible for the non-professional day-to-day administration and for routine maintenance and ordering. The administrator is usually supported by a team of secretaries. The management of this group may be delegated to her. Policies and procedures are discussed with all staff to reduce the non-teaching load of the teachers and fairly distribute the secretarial work.

The librarian and audio-visual aids technician have a vital supportive role. While these staff may be directly responsible to the Director of Nurse Education in many schools, the delegation of authority to a representative committee ensures that decisions related to use of resources and expenditure are agreed by all staff.

Financial management

The manager is charged with effective use of resources, people and time. Financial management involves forecasting expected expenditure, obtaining the necessary finances for that expenditure and monitoring it, with regard to both staff and non-staff.

In England, at present, financial resources for the school are obtained from two sources: the Health Authority and the Statutory Body.

The monies from the Health Authority include the salaries of learners undertaking a statutory training, those undertaking post-basic courses, teachers for the staff development team, personnel involved in selection and secretarial staff for these activities. Also included are the general overheads for running the school, rates, heating, etc., the cost involved in recruiting learners, the furniture and fittings and maintenance of the school and some stationery costs. All these have to be included in the bids made by the educational manager during the budget-fixing process of the Health Authority. In forecasting the budget, it is essential to bear in mind commitments already made to candidates for training in future years and to remember that adjustments may take over three years to work through the system. Financial resources for courses have to take account of fees and travelling expenses and require re-negotiating for each financial year.

Resources related to both the staff and equipment for basic nurse training are distributed by the Statutory Body via the Education Advisory Group. This Group, appointed by the English National Board for each Region, has within its terms of reference the disbursement of funds for basic nursing education. The director of nurse education is the named budget holder for these funds. Estimates are completed twice a year and forecasts take account of anticipated vacancies, those returning from or being seconded to courses and increases or reduction in learner numbers. Staff numbers are presently established on a 1:15 ratio. Other factors which might be considered include the number of school sites and the variety of training programmes. Non-staff resources are on a per capita basis plus a fixed sum for each school site.

Expenditure is monitored on a monthly basis when financial statements for each item of expenditure can be discussed with a financial adviser: such meetings provide the opportunity to discuss problems, progress and anticipated outcomes on a regular basis.

Evaluation

Evaluation of the school may include monitoring by the education officer of the Statutory Body and/or education board. It will include examination success rate, learner wastage and staff turnover and subjective evaluation such as the degree of job satisfaction and learning climate within the school.

Monitoring by the education officer occurs informally and less frequently on a formal basis with a full visit and report to the Statutory Body for continued approval. Changes in the format of training or assessment have to be discussed and approved by the Statutory Body. A Nurse Education Board may be formed at local level to receive reports concerning all aspects of nurse education and to monitor performance. Membership of this Board could include representatives from the employing authority, the Statutory Body, higher and further education, learners, nurse teachers, nurse managers and clinical nurses. An annual report of the activities of the school provides an additional monitoring mechanism.

Another aspect of the role of the manager of the school of nursing is liaison with external bodies, for example, colleges of further and higher education involved in all aspects of nurse education, particularly undergraduate nursing degree programmes and nurse teacher courses. The education manager is also one of the team of senior nurse managers in the Health Authority. This is discussed in the next section.

EDUCATIONAL MANAGEMENT WITHIN THE NURSING MANAGEMENT STRUCTURE

The majority of nurse education occurs within the National Health Service; the manager of education is part of the nursing management structure, and as such one of the nursing policy-making group. At present, the educational manager is directly responsible to the chief nursing officer. The role of the educational manager as part of this team is to contribute to policy-making and to assist in the management of the total nursing service of the Authority; the role is discussed in relation to the previously agreed components of management.

Planning

The planning system of the National Health Service will not be described in detail. A strategic plan for ten years has to be agreed by each Authority and a two-year operational plan agreed annually. The management of education in the planning cycle is to prepare the strategic and operational plan for nurse education and ensure educational courses to equip staff to meet the future service requirements included in the plan.

Educational planning involves identifying the skills and knowledge required by staff for the future services and providing means of acquiring these, either locally or by secondment to a suitable course. Courses planned at local level have to take account of cost, both in replacement staff and tutorial staff. Secondment costs time and money and these have to be balanced with the operational plan. Two-year plans have to take account of possible change, such as ratios of trained and untrained staff and external financial constraints. The educational manager involved in this planning can identify and discuss the effect of such change on the training programmes. The involvement of teachers in health care planning teams may enable the early identification of staff training needs for the services planned.

The policy-making group also decides aims for the nursing service and method of achieving them.

Organising

Organising the educational input into the nursing management structure involves organising the staff development programmes previously discussed. Additionally, it includes deciding the communication network which ensures that nurse managers, nurse educationalists and clinical nurses work in partnership to ensure the support of all nurse education programmes.

The partnership may be manifested by representatives from nursing management and nurse education being jointly involved in appointment of staff in each area. It is enhanced if they are specified liaison teachers for units of management at all levels, with access to each other's meetings as appropriate. Formal meetings included in the communication network include the curriculum development group, assessment meetings, nursing practice groups and others agreed locally. The organisation of a formal committee structure within a Health Authority provides the opportunity for the educational manager to participate in policy-making as it affects the total nursing service.

Leading

Within the nursing management structure, the educational manager has a role as a resource person, sharing with colleagues professional awareness and initiating discussions on professional issues. The role comprises identifying research findings which may be implemented in nursing practice or areas for further research; motivating individuals within the organisation through their immediate managers to fulfil their potential and make use of the educational opportunities available to them; and agreeing with the policy-making team the programme of staff development and methods for measuring its effectiveness.

Controlling

Educational management within the National Health Service is concerned with controlling the standard of care and the learning environment. Methods for control include the monitoring of sickness/absence in each clinical area and the monitoring of complaints and incidents and discussing these with appropriate service managers to identify possible causes and initiate remedies. Monitoring also includes agreeing criteria for assessing nursing practice, including the process, environment and outcome of nursing actions. Measuring standards of care is not easy, but it is suggested that some criteria may be agreed which can then be monitored: the incidence of wound infection and pressure sores are possible indicators. Monitoring the effect of new policies and their implementation against the workload of staff and demands of learners is also necessary.

The management of education involves ensuring that initial training programmes meet the needs of learners and the requirements of the Statutory Body and ensure a service to patients. It includes managing post-basic opportunities and staff development programmes. The management of the school and teaching staff and the educational input as a part of the total nursing management structure have also been considered. Nursing and the Health Service are in a state of flux. It is essential that the management of nurse education enables the development of safe, competent practitioners who accept professional responsibility for their continuing education to ensure a sound knowledge base for future professional practice.

Suggested further reading

Fretwell, J. (1982) *Ward Teaching & Learning*. London: Royal College of Nursing.
Ogier, M. (1982) *An Ideal Sister*. London: Royal College of Nursing.
Orton, H.D. (1981) *Ward Learning Climate*. London: Royal College of Nursing.
Stenhouse, L. (1975) *An Introduction to Curriculum Research and Development*. London: Heinemann.

Chapter 9
Managing the Profession

REGINALD PYNE

It may be fortuitous, but this book is being written at a time when the statutory framework of the nursing profession is undergoing its most significant change since the passage into law of the Nurses Registration Act of 1919. Whether another 60 years will elapse before any further major change in the area of legislation that affects and regulates the profession, it is impossible to know. What is certain, however, is that the new structure will apply for a sufficient period of time to have an influence on the professional lives of several generations of nurses.

It is, therefore, important that nurses should understand the law and the statutory structure concerned with the profession's preparation and regulation. For the nurse aspiring to be a professional manager such an understanding is essential, and failure to possess it would alone constitute a good reason for rejecting an application for a middle management post. That may, at first sight, appear to be an extreme and arrogant statement. I hope that further consideration will result in agreement that it is an accurate one. After all, what is involved is a new piece of legislation that provides the structure within which we are meant to ensure a number of important things for the future. This law is concerned with how members of the nursing profession achieve professional competence in the first place, how they maintain their competence, how they increase their competence and (hopefully) approach and achieve excellence, and how they may lose the right to practise if (for any of several reasons) they cease to be competent. In short, it is about the protection of the often vulnerable public we exist to serve.

It is, however, important before looking in greater depth at the new law that we take a brief glance at the past. This is necessary because a great many nurses will have become familiar with the existence and roles of a number of statutory bodies which no longer exist. It is also necessary in order that the past achievements of those statutory bodies (operating as they were within the constraints of outdated legislation that increasingly limited rather than enabled them in certain areas of their work) may be recognised. We should certainly note that, for more than a decade, these statutory bodies drew attention to the inadequacies of the law they had to operate. They, like the Committee on Nursing (chaired by Lord Briggs), and in company with the major professional organisations and many articulate individuals within the profession, are to be thanked for the fact that we have new legislation on the statute book and now in operation in the form of the Nurses, Midwives and Health Visitors Act 1979.

It is this Act of Parliament that created a new structure – one which draws the preparation and regulation of nurses, midwives and health visitors into one coordinated system for the first time, one which lays before the members of the profession the challenge of improving that preparation and regulation in the interests of the public. But first, and in order to achieve that objective, the Act (by the repeal of a number of earlier Acts of Parliament) had to bring to an end the separate existence of a number of statutory bodies. These were:

1. The General Nursing Council for England and Wales
2. The General Nursing Council for Scotland
3. The Northern Ireland Council for Nurses and Midwives
4. The Central Midwives Board (for England and Wales)
5. The Central Midwives Board for Scotland
6. The Council for the Education and Training of Health Visitors

With the exception of the last of these, whose functions were explained by its title, the statutory bodies named were responsible in law for controlling admission to their registers, for maintaining publicly accessible records (so that those who needed to know could ascertain the names, etc. of those from whom competent professional care might be expected), for prosecuting or arranging the prosecution of those who falsely claimed statutory professional qualifications, and for taking appropriate action against those who were proved to be guilty of misconduct in a professional sense, including (where necessary) removing them from the registers.

The Nurses, Midwives and Health Visitors Act 1979 also brought to an end the independent existence of three other organisations, not by repealing yet more Acts of Parliament (since these were not bodies introduced by statute), but by placing responsibility for their former work of specialist post-basic training within the new statutory structure. These three organisations were:

1. The Joint Board of Clinical Nursing Studies
2. The Committee for Clinical Nursing Studies
3. The Panel of Assessors for District Nurse Training

Thus, the new Act cleared the way for a coordinated approach to preparation and regulation in the nursing, midwifery and health visiting professions.

The new statutory structure can appear horrendously complicated, but so (it must be remembered) was that which it replaced. In the past, there were nine separate and independent organisations with either no, or at best minimal, overlap of membership. In spite of their best efforts, it was not always possible to ensure a cohesive approach or to work to apply collective pressure on matters of important professional concern. The new statutory structure improves on that of the past in several important respects. One such respect is that the new statutory bodies are, in effect, made creatures one of another by virtue of the fact that the Act requires each of the four national bodies (the National Boards for Nursing, Midwifery and Health Visiting) to appoint seven of its members to also serve as members of the United Kingdom body (the United Kingdom Central Council for Nursing, Midwifery and Health Visiting, or UKCC), where together they form a majority. A further, and surely highly important, factor is that the members of the professions themselves, through a democratic election process, choose two out of each three national board members, and thus 102 of the 168 members, of this integrated structure of professional control.

The Nurses, Midwives and Health Visitors Act 1979, in common with other sections of the law concerning the professions, does not set down every function to be performed by the statutory bodies. It states their principal functions, or indicates what those functions shall include. This can generally be taken to mean that, provided an Act does not state that a statutory body definitely cannot do a certain thing, it is understood that (if it so chooses) it can, always providing it accords with the spirit of the legislation, falls within the general parameters prescribed, and deals with obviously relevant matters.

The Act provided for the establishment of a body called the United Kingdom Central Council for Nursing, Midwifery and Health Visiting (with a membership described in outline in Figure 4) or UKCC. The principal functions of the Council are stated in section 2 of the Nurses, Midwives and Health Visitors Act 1979 in the following terms:

1. The principal functions of the Central Council shall be to establish and improve standards of training and professional conduct for nurses, midwives and health visitors.
2. The Council shall ensure that the standards of training they establish are such as to meet any (European) Community obligation of the United Kingdom.
3. The Council shall by means of rules determine the conditions of a person's being admitted to training, and the kind and standard of training to be undertaken with a view to registration.

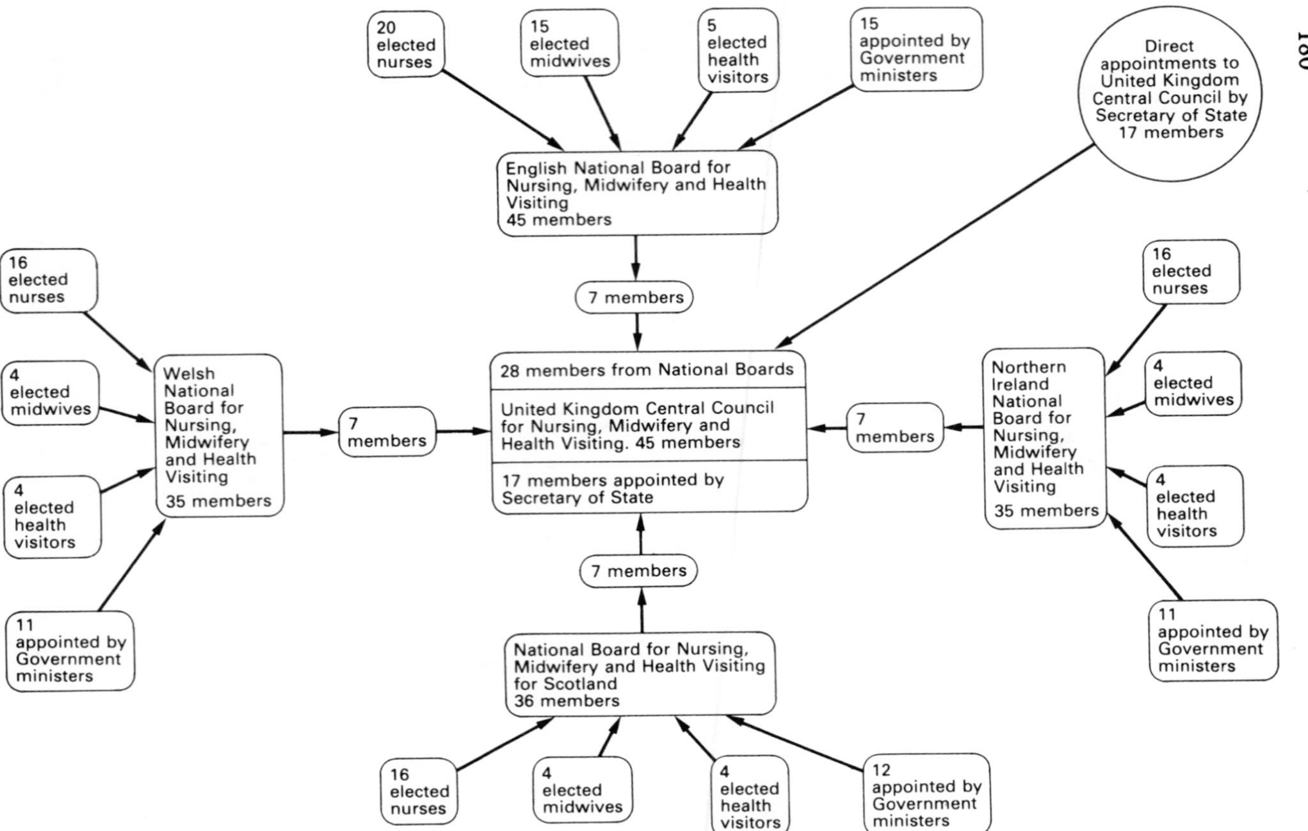

Figure 4. The United Kingdom Central Council for Nursing, Midwifery and Health Visiting.

4. The rules may also make provision with respect to the kind and standard of further training available to persons who are already registered.
5. The powers of the Council shall include that of providing, in such manner as it thinks fit, advice for nurses, midwives and health visitors on standards of professional conduct.
6. In the discharge of its functions the Council shall have proper regard for the interests of all groups within the professions, including those with minority representation.

Some elaboration upon that section of the Act is needed. A careful reading of it reveals a number of points.

1. The Council is required to 'make rules' as a means of achieving certain things. This simply means that it determines those features that it wishes to include in subordinate legislation (more law, but in the form of statutory instruments rather than an Act), instructs its lawyers to state its intentions in legal terminology, and then in some cases places them before Parliament for approval, and in others submits them for the approval of ministers. Rule-making is the means by which flesh is put on the skeleton which is the basic enabling Act.
2. It states the 'principal functions of the Central Council' in important but general terms, leaving the Council to work out how it will meet these key objectives. By referring to the 'principal functions' it does not exclude others. Indeed, certain other functions of the Council are clearly prescribed in sections 10, 11 and 12 of the Act. Reference to these sections is included later in the chapter.
3. It is exciting and at least potentially revolutionary in its requirements (note the use of the word 'shall') that the Council 'shall improve standards of training and professional conduct'.
4. Next, this legislation is important because it brings 'further training' firmly within the statutory professional framework where it has not been hitherto.
5. The use of the word 'shall' in the sub-section requiring the Council to give advice on standards of professional conduct faces the Council at one and the same time with an interesting challenge and a tremendous responsibility. At the same time it seems to introduce an overtly (even if unintended) 'political' element into the situation, for it seems to be difficult if not impossible to advise on standards of professional conduct without taking note of and being influenced by the pressures of the work-place which provides the context in which the professionals concerned do their work.

An implicit corollary to the requirement of the Act that advice be given so as to improve standards of conduct is a responsibility to draw attention to the fact when pressures (arising from matters outside the Council's control) obstruct the achievement of the required improvement. Another is that the advice that is given should indicate to practitioners what their profession expects of them, and, while not stating what things might constitute misconduct, provides the base against which conduct can be measured.

Section 5(1) of the Act requires that 'England, Wales, Scotland and Northern Ireland shall each have a National Board for Nursing, Midwifery and Health Visiting, and, the Boards shall be corporate bodies'. Section 6 prescribes the functions of the Boards in the following terms:

(1) The National Boards shall in England, Wales, Scotland and Northern Ireland respectively –
(a) provide, or arrange for others to provide, at institutions approved by the Board –
  (i) courses of training with a view to enabling persons to qualify for registration as nurses, midwives or health visitors or for the recording of additional qualifications in the register; and
  (ii) courses of further training for those already registered;
(b) ensure that such courses meet the requirements of the Central Council as to their content and standard;
(c) hold, or arrange for others to hold, such examinations as are necessary to enable persons to satisfy requirements for registration or to obtain additional qualifications;
(d) collaborate with the Council in the promotion of improved training methods; and
(e) carry out investigations of cases of alleged misconduct, with a view to proceedings before the Central Council or a committee of the Council for a person to be removed from the register.
(2) The National Boards shall discharge their functions subject to and in accordance with any applicable rules of the Council and shall have proper regard for the interests of all groups within the professions, including those with minority representation.

In most of its sub-sections, section 6 of the Act is very specific indeed. It leaves no room for doubt that the Boards have a major executive function to perform in respect of all that is concerned with education, training and examinations. It is, however, equally clear that they must fulfil their responsibilities within the parameters, and in accordance with the principles determined by the Central Council. This is, therefore, a positive clause, in that it accepts that there can be a variety of routes to the same destination, and allows for useful variation and experiment while recognising that in the end the products of the preparation will be admitted to the one central professional register.

The Nurses, Midwives and Health Visitors Act passed into law in 1979 in literally the last hour of the last day of an outgoing Parliament, and in the run up to a General Election. Although the Act had not been the subject of party dissension, it was several months later, and following further waves of pressure from the professions, that the Secretary of State brought forward an Order to implement its first phases with effect from September 1980. This order constituted the National Boards and Central Council with an all-appointed membership for the first three years of their existence. During this initial three years, at the end of which the bodies would be reconstituted and possess a significant elected component, the new bodies were to exist in overlap with the old. In effect, therefore, the statutory and training bodies which were to be phased out in 1983 were left until then bearing responsibility for the tasks placed upon them by earlier legislation (training, examinations, registration, professional discipline, etc.). During the same time, the Central Council and National Boards had to concentrate on preparing the future.

This preparation had to concentrate on two separate yet related areas of activity. First, while accepting that they had to start from where the phasing out organisations were (and inherit their workload, range of courses, etc.), they also had to determine how they would approach the task of satisfying the requirements of the Act in the future. Secondly, they had to prepare committee structures that would facilitate their subsequent work in a positive, dynamic manner.

The Central Council were faced with an additional task during the overlap period. Not only does the Act require it to 'make rules' in respect of many specific issues and 'for the purpose of giving effect to this Act'. Section 22(3) of the Act also requires the Council, before making any rules, to consult 'representatives of any groups of persons who appear likely to be affected by the proposed rules'. This is an interesting new feature of legislation concerning the nursing, midwifery and health visiting professions, and surely a positive one. It is important to note that it is a requirement that was not simply for the initial policy determination and rule-making phase, but one which continues to apply until the Act (or at least the relevant part of it) is repealed.

The existence of this clause led to the production of some interesting and stimulating consultation papers by Working Groups composed of Central Council and National Board members during the first half of the three-year overlap period. These consultation papers were aimed at stimulating serious consideration of the issues they raised and at producing constructive responses which would assist the determination of policies on key issues. They were, therefore, distributed very widely so as to draw forth views not only from those within the professions affected, but from related professions and from groups who could represent consumer interest.

Five specific issues became the subject of consultation papers from the Council during the period in which it was preparing to make the first statutory rules. The first concerned a proposed scheme by which a majority of members of National Boards would be elected by their professional peers in 1983. The second discussed the Single Professional Register that the Act required to replace the various statutory forms of records of the bodies which ceased to exist in 1983, and certain major associated issues. The third was a broad-based, philosophical paper which raised a number of long-term questions about basic nursing education, including the possible eventual phasing out of training for a second level of nurse qualification. The fourth was prepared for the purpose of explaining the ways in which the nursing and midwifery professions had been subject to professional disciplinary control in the past, and for making proposals concerning the future 'professional conduct' mechanism and several important allied matters. The fifth Working Group was concerned with recommending initial committee structures for the Council. In all cases, the consultation papers became the subject of discussion and debate throughout the United Kingdom, and produced the volume of response that clearly indicated a welcome for this new procedure. It is one of the ways in which those in the clinical situation can have an effect upon the determination of future professional policies.

The residue of this chapter is concerned primarily with the authority that lies within the statutory structure to remove nurses, midwives and health visitors from that register or part(s) of it, and to restore to all or part(s) of the register persons who have previously been removed. It also sets out to outline, explain and comment upon the legislation, structure and procedures through which this function of the new statutory bodies is performed in the public interest. But before doing any of these things, it is necessary to elaborate upon the second and third of the consultation papers referred to above, since certain of the issues the originating members raised (using the new and positive demands of the Nurses, Midwives and Health Visitors Act to advantage) underlay and have done much to determine subsequent developments.

The Working Group (convened by the UKCC from within its own membership and the National Boards) given the remit of considering how the required 'Single Professional Register' and its levels and parts could first be created and then maintained, and recommending the policies that should apply to that maintenance were faced with an interesting and challenging task.

Its members recognised the inadequacies of previous legislation which, with the exception of that concerning midwifery, simply required an assessment of competence at the completion of training and as a prelude to registration, but no subsequent updating of knowledge or assessment of competence in order to retain registration status. They regarded that situation as unsatisfactory. They took the view that it was completely illogical to draw nursing, midwifery and health visiting into one coordinated system of statutory control without requiring a move for all into the ground that midwifery had long occupied. The midwifery profession had operated around the principle, set down in statutory rules, that a qualified midwife, even if in continuous practice, could not continue so to practise unless, each five years, she attended a mandatory refresher course. If she did not attend and complete such a course, her right to practise expired. Although there has not been universal approval for the content of those courses, the principle was clearly sound and deserving of wider application.

The same Working Group's members also noted (from the records of the outgoing bodies' professional disciplinary work) that the former statutory bodies not infrequently found themselves using the awesome power of their professional disciplinary machinery to deal with situations that would not have arisen had the law required an updating of knowledge, skill and competence before allowing qualified people to return to practice after a break of several years.

The concerns they felt on these matters were a feature of the Group's Consultation Paper which was widely distributed for comment early in 1982. The rather different proposals it made for the future received widespread and enthusiastic support, despite the fact that this support came from a profession of which more would consequently be asked so as to allow continued eligibility to practise. The Working Group, and subsequently the United Kingdom Central Council in accepting its recommendations as being in the public interest, could therefore be seen as having a substantial mandate from the nursing, midwifery and health visiting professions.

Thus, there are plans for the future to carry into subordinate legislation (through the making of statutory rules) a provision whereby a person who has been out of professional practice for five years or more must attend a form of retraining/refresher course before being permitted to practise again. Also in the future, as soon as resources make it possible, it is planned that it will become a requirement that those in practice must, in order to retain that right, re-register periodically. That renewal of registration will become dependent on (for example) attendance at a mandatory course, or evidence of recent further or continuing professional education/updating. Also at some future stage, there are plans to introduce a maximum age for professional practice which may only be exceeded with the express permission of the UKCC.

These measures, especially when allied to the creation of a single professional register to which employers of nurses, midwives and health visitors can have access to ascertain a person's range of qualifications and eligibility to practise from one source, are surely in the public interest. They will also be consistent with the sections of the Nurses, Midwives and Health Visitors Act that require the Council to effect improvements, give advice on standards of professional conduct, and make alterations to entries in the register.

The other Consultation Paper to which I must refer in some detail was produced by a similarly convened Working Group whose terms of reference required them to consider those parts of the Act concerned with removal from or restoration to the register, and allied matters. This group's Consultation Paper was also widely distributed, and stimulated healthy and constructive discussion of an often misunderstood or almost taboo subject. It also was warmly welcomed and comprehensively supported by the profession, and therefore gave the UKCC a positive mandate to introduce from the outset, through statutory rules, the structures which are fully described in the following pages.

Before dealing with the new rules, and the structures and procedures that have been created as a result of their form, it is necessary to take another look back so that the reader may see how the new differs from the old. The crucial difference lies in the fact that while the repealed Acts, under which the Nursing Councils and Midwifery Boards existed, referred to and allowed removal from the respective registers for 'misconduct', the Nurses, Midwives and Health Visitors Act uses those same words but then adds 'or otherwise'.

Previously, the statutory bodies were in considerable difficulty in fulfilling their role as protectors of the public, since they had to await the occurrence of some culpable act which they might then consider misconduct before taking action. On many occasions this has resulted in members of the nursing and midwifery professions continuing in practice when illness was robbing them of insight, and debilitating their competence and safety. Then, when an incident (sometimes a tragic incident) eventually occurred on which action could be taken, the awesome disciplinary system was used to protect the public from a person whose 'offence' was basically that he or she was ill.

(I have previously commented upon this at length in *Professional Discipline in Nursing – Theory and Practice.*)

It must be assumed that the drafters of the new legislation had heard the anguished expressions of concern from members and staff of the former bodies about the inadequacy of that which it has replaced. Although the new Act does not specify anything other than 'misconduct' as grounds for removal from the register, it opened the door so that members (in developing statutory rules' content) could determine other grounds for removal. The positive opportunities provided by the insertion of the words 'or otherwise' were ventilated in the Consultation Paper, and the response made it clear that the profession shared the concern of the former bodies, and endorsed the proposal of the UKCC Working Group to use those opportunities. Evidence of such professional support assisted the Council when the time came for it to determine its policies as a prelude to the drafting of rules. The resultant policies are reflected in the procedures which are stated and elaborated upon in later paragraphs.

Since the Consultation Paper on this subject was so warmly welcomed by the professions concerned, it would be remiss of me not to reproduce from it the section which set out to define professional misconduct, and then to elaborate upon that definition:

(a) The Exercise of Professional Discipline – What it is

(i) It is the statutory bodies concerned with nursing, midwifery and health visiting exercising their role as protectors of the public;

(ii) it is an integral part of fulfilling the role of ensuring the maintenance of professional standards.

(b) The Exercise of Professional Discipline – What it is not

(i) it is not its purpose to punish;
NOTE: In this respect it is recognised that removal from the Register following a hearing might be construed as punishment. This, or any other course of action, is however aimed at protecting the public and is not, and should not be regarded as being a punitive measure.

(ii) it is not a means whereby nurse managers or health authorities can solve their management/employment problems.

Within the context of (a) and (b) above, it can also result in, or be a contribution to, the rehabilitation of the persons concerned against whom action has been taken.

In the light of its considerations of points made by respondents, the Working Group, when making its recommendations to Council, extended the 'Comment' that concludes that extract by adding the following sentence: 'It can also be the means by which members of the professions can publicly clear their names when they are the subject of unfounded allegations.' The Working Group's elaboration of its definition was also welcomed. For this reason, and because (like the definition) it is basic material on which the recommendations were built, it also was restated in the Group's report to the Council.

The Positive Role
The positive role is encompassed within the definition in (a) above, i.e. protection of the public, maintenance of professional standards; when individual cases are considered, they invariably overlap. It is the first, protecting the public, which should be seen as paramount although the way in which this function is exercised makes it possible to contribute to the other.

The Negative Role
Experience also suggests that the negative definitions as set out in paragraph (b) above need to be discussed since there continues to be a great deal of misunderstanding and confusion between the maintenance of standards of professional conduct and punishment.

The Criminal Courts exist to deal with those who break the law. It is, on the other hand, for the professions, through their statutory bodies, to decide whether an offence for which an individual nurse, midwife or health visitor, has been convicted is such that it might constitute professional misconduct and should therefore result in the matter being processed through the disciplinary machinery to reach a determination as to whether the name of the convicted person should be removed from the professional Register.

The Working Group considers that it is essential to differentiate between the 'disciplinary' role of the employer and that of the statutory bodies. The former relates to the nurse, midwife or health visitor as an employee who has offended in some way which affects her role as an employee. The difficult decision as to whether employment should be continued, is a management decision. The role of the statutory bodies is concerned with the individual nurse, midwife or health visitor as a professional person rather than as an employee and relates to consideration as to whether certain conduct of an individual constitutes professional misconduct. In these circumstances, the statutory body must give consideration as to whether the conduct was of such a nature as to warrant removal from the Register.

The two aspects of discipline outlined above may be interrelated in the sense that a misdemeanour which warrants disciplinary action in the employment situation may be such as to be considered also as professional misconduct; this is not however invariably so. It would be wrong therefore for either management or the statutory body to await the outcome of the decision by the other before taking action appropriate to their respective role.

It is important that members of the profession should remember their individual responsibility to report to the relevant statutory body any misdemeanour on the part of a nurse, midwife or health visitor which in their professional judgement constitutes professional misconduct.

What has emerged from this consideration of and consultation about the problems of the past and the opportunities provided by the Nurses,

Midwives and Health Visitors Act 1979? The answer is that in two quite significant respects the UKCC has broken new ground. It has done this by taking a first major step towards fulfilling its obligations under section 2(5) of the Act by introducing a document entitled *Code of Professional Conduct for Nurses, Midwives and Health Visitors*. This document, now being issued to all who are newly admitted to any part of the professional register of nurses, midwives and health visitors, and also through a variety of channels to those whose names already feature in the register, seeks to advise practitioners of the basic principles which should underlie their conduct.

The second means by which the UKCC has broken new ground is seen in the fact that it has used its rule-making powers to introduce what (for nursing, midwifery and health visiting) is a totally new procedure through which it can question the right to practise of those who are alleged to be unsafe practitioners because they are ill. These rules have been made under section 12(1) of the Act which allows for removal for misconduct *or otherwise*.

Before going into further detail about this or the mechanism through which questions of possible professional misconduct are considered, it seems wise to consider the *Code of Professional Conduct* in more detail. The reason for this is found in the fact that, through its 12 points based on ethical concepts and through several associated statements, it does a number of things.

The text of this important document reads as follows:

The registered nurse, midwife or health visitor shall, at all times, act in such a manner as to justify public trust and confidence, to uphold and enhance the good standing and reputation of the profession, to serve the public interest and the interests of patients/clients.

In fulfilment of professional responsibility and in the exercise of professional accountability the nurse, midwife or health visitor shall:

1. Comply with the law of any country, state, province or territory in which she works, and have due regard to custom and practice.
2. Be accountable for her practice and take every reasonable opportunity to sustain and improve her knowledge and professional competence.
3. Have regard to the customs, values and spiritual beliefs of patients/clients.
4. Hold in confidence any information obtained through professional attendance on a patient/client. Such information must not be divulged unless judged necessary to discharge her professional responsibilities to the patient/client; normally the consent of the patient/client should be obtained. Exceptionally the professional practitioner may be required by legal process to divulge information held: she should seek advice before responding.
5. Avoid any abuse of the privileged relationship with patients/clients or the privileged access to their property, residence or workplace.

6. At all times act in such a way as to promote and safeguard the well being and interests of patients/clients for whose care she is professionally accountable and ensure that by no action or omission on her part their condition or safety is placed at risk.
7. Have regard to the environment of care (physical, psychological and social) and to available resources, and make known to the appropriate authority if these endanger safe standards of practice.
8. Accept a responsibility relevant to her professional experience for assisting her peers and subordinates to develop professional competence.
9. Have due regard to the workload of and the pressures on professional colleagues and subordinates and take appropriate action if these are seen to be such as to endanger safe standards of practice.
10. Make known to the appropriate authority any conscientious objection she holds which may be relevant to her professional practice.
11. Refuse to accept any gift, favour or hospitality which might be interpreted as seeking to exert undue influence to obtain preferential treatment.
12. Avoid advertising or signing an advertisement using her professional qualification(s) to encourage the sale of commercial products, or services. Any nurse, midwife or health visitor who wishes to use her professional qualifications to advertise her professional services or to take part in any form of commercial advertising should seek advice at the UKCC offices.

Notes associated with the document indicate that to challenge what is considered an unsatisfactory law through the due processes of democracy, or unsound practices through appropriate professional channels, is regarded by the UKCC as a proper expression of professional concern and responsibility. Further to that, it is made clear that the document is intended to be dynamic and relevant to the social and professional context in which nurses, midwives and health visitors practise, and requires that practitioners enter into dialogue with the UKCC to facilitate its review and updating.

It can readily be seen from even a cursory reading that the *Code of Professional Conduct* emphasises for practitioners that, just as the Nurses, Midwives and Health Visitors Act (and the statutory rules made under its powers) places the interests of the public (when at their most vulnerable) first, so must they. Thus, there are four points which directly concern patients, and another which, by referring to 'the environment of care', is concerned with safe standards of practice.

It can also be seen that the individual's accountability for his or her practice, and responsibility for maintaining and improving both knowledge and competence, are emphasised. This is not to be done as a matter of academic interest, but because it clearly goes to the subject of standards of care.

All these points, together with that which requires compliance with the law, underlie the subject of professional misconduct, what it is, and how it is to be evaluated. But the *Code* also contains two points which are concerned with the responsibility we have for and to colleagues. Failure in these respects might also form the basis of allegations of misconduct. In this context the more senior your position the greater your responsibility, and therefore the greater your vulnerability if you fail to properly fulfil those responsibilities. The points concerning colleagues must also have an obvious relevance to the issue of fitness to practise with which the UKCC has concerned itself.

Recognition of the latter point led the UKCC to introduce a new structure and procedures, the purpose of which is to consider those cases wherein it is suggested that a nurse, midwife or health visitor is unfit to practise because she is ill, and thus endangers her patients. Brief reference has already been made to these new procedures introduced by subordinate legislation. More detailed explanation and comment follows an elaboration of the machinery to consider issues of professional misconduct, since it is from the committees wielding powers within that machinery that a considerable number of referrals into the 'fitness to practise' channel come.

Turning, then, to a more detailed explanation of the new procedures for dealing with allegations of misconduct first involves reminding the reader that section 6(1)(e) of the Nurses, Midwives and Health Visitors Act requires that: 'The National Boards ... shall carry out investigations of cases of alleged misconduct with a view to proceedings before the Central Council or a committee of the Council for a person to be removed from the register.' The Act also requires the Boards to: '... discharge their functions subject to and in accordance with any applicable rules of the Council and ... have proper regard for the interests of all groups within the profession, including those with minority representation'.

The 'applicable rules of the Council' in the context now referred to are relatively few. What they require of the Boards is as follows:

1. That they shall carry out investigations of cases of alleged misconduct by practitioners who are normally resident in their respective territories and which have been referred to them direct or through the Council.
2. That the Committee of the Board which considers such matters shall not include any members who at the same time are UKCC members and thus might have to hear the same matters at a subsequent and more serious stage.
3. That any practitioner who is alleged to be guilty of misconduct shall be told of the fact and invited to submit a written statement or explanation for consideration by the Board committee.
4. That the Board, through its officers or solicitor, shall gather all relevant

reports and information to enable its committee to make a considered collective professional judgement on the matters placed before it.

5. That the committee shall consider whether any case is one which justifies a hearing before the Professional Conduct Committee of the Council with a view to that practitioner being removed from the register or any part or parts of it, and shall resolve accordingly.
6. That, should the committee in the course of its deliberations form the opinion that things alleged may be a consequence of or indication of illness, they should refer the case to the Health Committee of the Council.

These requirements apply irrespective of the source from which a case is received. There are three main sources (Figure 5). That there are three main

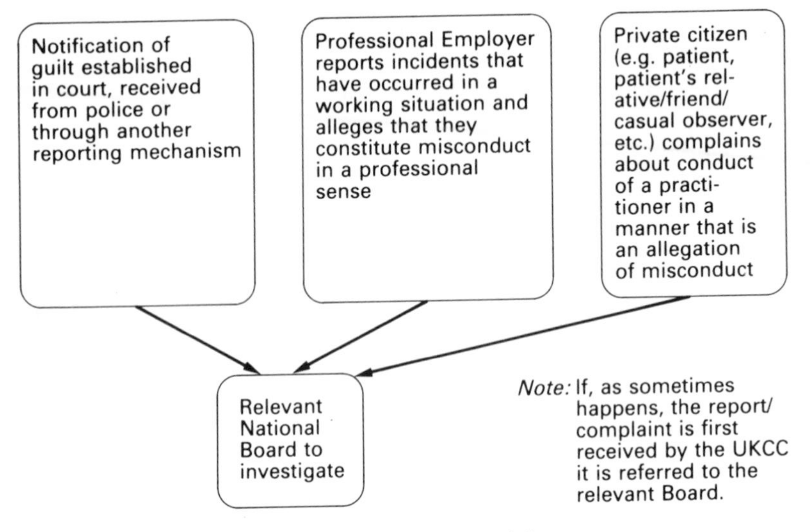

Figure 5. Sources of complaint.

sources of report is important, and needs to be recognised. The fact that a manager chooses not to bring a complaint to a Board does not mean that it will not be made. Staff more junior to that manager have the same rights in these matters, as do any private citizens. Irrespective of the source of a complaint, the Board have a responsibility in law to investigate it thoroughly. The procedures they follow to achieve this where the case emanates from a finding of guilt in a criminal court are outlined in Figure 6.

Where the report involves a person who is not the subject of guilt established in a criminal court, but rather of complaint from an employer or

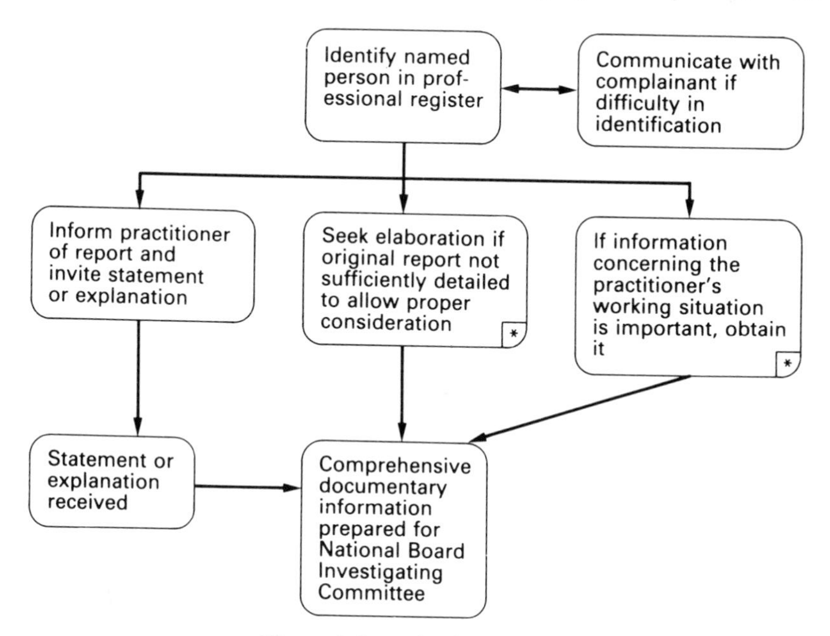

Figure 6. Investigation procedure.

private citizen, the situation is different. Here you are dealing with what, at the report stage, are not established facts but unproven allegations. Unless the information is so comprehensive and well prepared as to render it unnecessary, the relevant Board officers will instruct the solicitor to visit the location concerned, to interview and take statements from any witnesses to the incidents described. This is necessary in order that the Board Investigating Committee should be sufficiently informed to be able to make a sound judgement. It is also essential that the evidence be thoroughly tested since the witnesses in question will (if the case is referred for a hearing with a view to possible removal from the register) have to give that evidence in person and be cross-examined by the respondent's representative, and questioned by the Professional Conduct Committee. In investigating a case, the solicitor also gathers information concerning any local arrangements or policies (for example, a local policy document on the control and administration of drugs) which is germane to the allegations under review. (With the substitution of these activities for those in the boxes marked with the symbol [*], Figure 6 is also valid for this category of cases.)

The Investigating Committee of each National Board has a serious and very significant role. It does not have the advantage of meeting the individual practitioner whose life and career it is considering. Its decision has to be made on the basis of documentary evidence which, in spite of the efforts of the officers and solicitor, will not always be as comprehensive as was hoped. It is not in its power to label any matter as misconduct, but it must form an opinion as to whether the matters under consideration are such as may possibly constitute misconduct before arriving at a decision. The small range of decisions available to the Investigating Committee might suggest that its powers are very limited. Note, however, that it has the awesome power to decide that matters reported to it shall not be forwarded for a hearing at which the question of removal from the register would have been an issue. The range of decisions available to the Investigating Committee are indicated in Figure 7. Whichever of them applies, the person concerned must be notified.

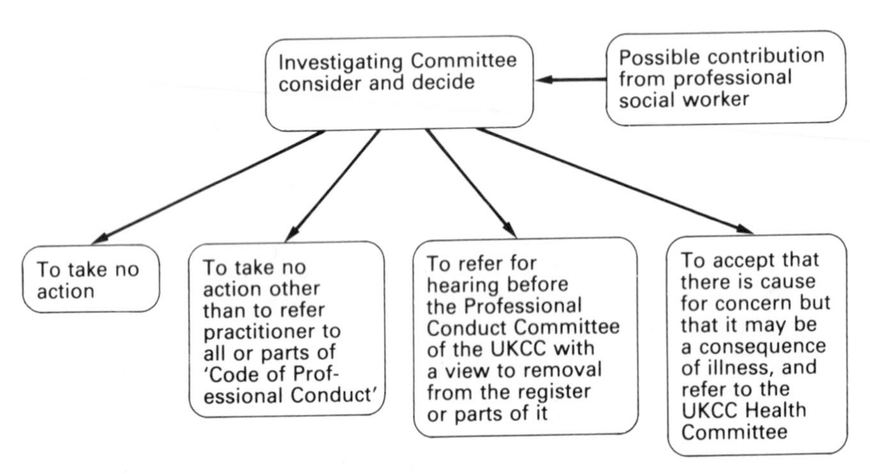

Figure 7. Decisions available to Investigating Committee.

In consequence of the gathering and careful consideration of evidence, information and opinion referred to above, a substantial number of those people who are the subject of reports or complaints are not referred to either of the UKCC committees for consideration. Instead, they are told that the matters are not being referred, although some advice may be given by reference to the *Code*.

The volume of cases to be considered by the committees of the UKCC is, therefore, substantially less than the original number reported by the Boards. The reason for this is that the predominantly nurse/midwife/health visitor members of the Investigating Committees, acting as a professional sieve, have rejected those matters which are not of professional concern, or at least not of such concern as to put the registration status of the people concerned at risk.

The two committees of the UKCC therefore are involved with much smaller numbers of practitioners and incidents, but invariably those that are of fairly obvious professional concern. More detail of the procedures concerned with the question of fitness to practise is given later. First, attention is drawn to the role and work of the UKCC Professional Conduct Committee.

Use of the word 'committee' is a little misleading in this context since it suggests a small number of members drawn from a larger body or organisation. In this case, the statutory rules require that all (45) members of the UKCC must be members of the Professional Conduct Committee, and that a minimum of five members must be assembled to constitute the committee to consider any case referred to it for hearing. It is also important to note that both the Act and the statutory rules make the point very strongly that the committee convened to adjudicate upon a person's conduct must be constituted '... with due regard to the professional field in which the respondent works or has worked'. This important clause in the new legislation renders it different from that which it replaces. It is clearly important, not only because midwives and health visitors are subject to the same regulatory powers as nurses, but also in order that practitioners from the specialisations within nursing may know that they are being appropriately judged.

Where a person has been referred by the committee of a National Board for a hearing, the end-result of which may be removal of the right to practise, the officers of the UKCC, in arranging that hearing, must satisfy the law in a number of important respects. Not only must they convene a specific committee 'with due regard to the professional field', etc. They must also satisfy the law in respect of due notice of the hearing, and ensure that the respondent is made aware of his or her right to appear in person, and to be represented by any barrister, solicitor, officer of a professional organisation or trade union, friend or relative.

Before elaborating upon the procedures of the Professional Conduct Committee, it is necessary to introduce some explanation of the term 'misconduct', since it has already been used a number of times, and must inevitably be used many more. The Act only uses the word when stating one of the functions of the National Boards ('to carry out investigations of cases of alleged misconduct'), and when requiring the UKCC to make statutory rules determining 'circumstances in which, and the means by which a person may, for misconduct or otherwise, be removed from the register or part of it ...'.

The Professional Conduct Rules (Statutory Instrument 1983, No. 887) themselves introduce a certain amount of clarification. The interpretation clause in the section includes the following definition: 'Misconduct means conduct unworthy of a nurse, midwife or health visitor as the case may be'. A later passage of text (in the part of the rules concerned with procedure at the Professional Conduct Committee) makes it clear that even proof of conviction in a criminal court does not of itself constitute misconduct – it is just a piece of evidence to consider before determining whether a particular misdemeanour is misconduct. In other words, nothing is misconduct in this specifically professional sense until a committee primarily composed of relevant professionals says it is, and they arrive at the point of making such a decision only after first satisfying themselves that guilt has been established in the ways illustrated in Figures 8 and 9.

Figure 8 is concerned with those cases in which the basis for the case is that the person has been convicted of a crime in a criminal court in the United

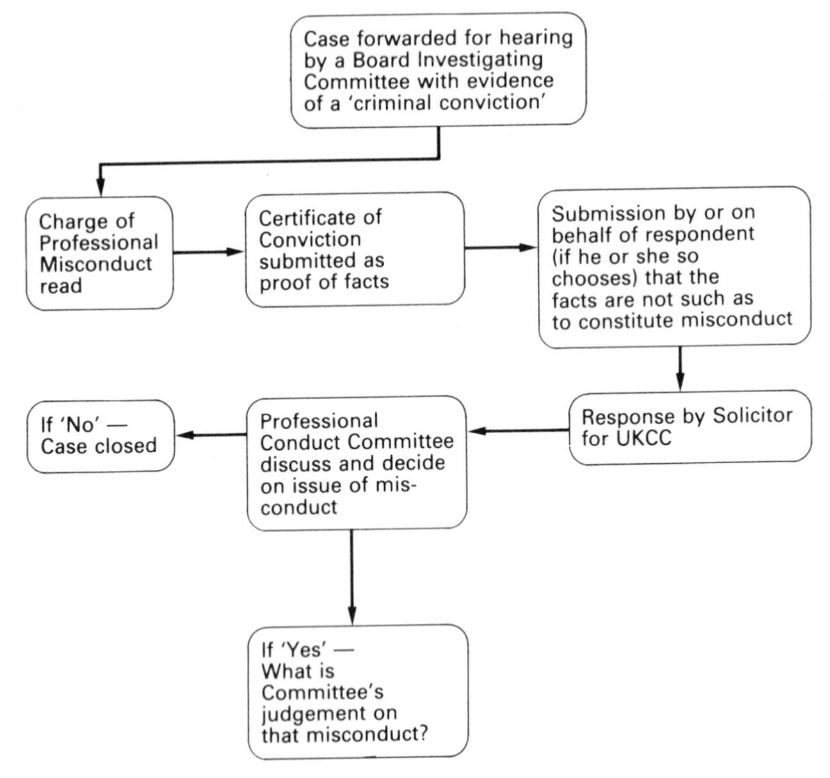

Figure 8. Establishment of guilt in cases of criminal conviction.

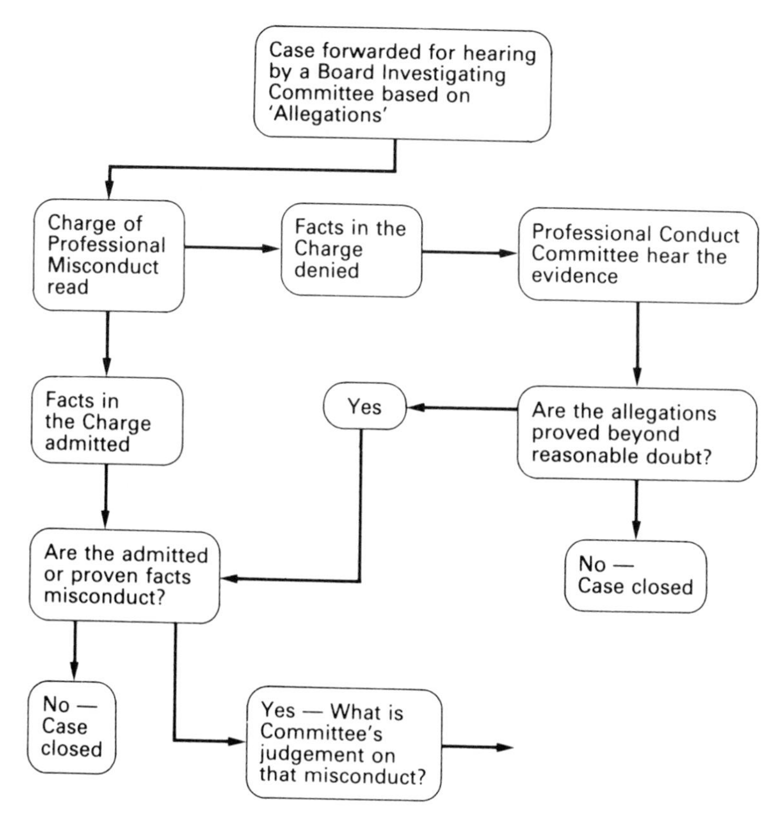

Figure 9. Establishment of guilt in cases of 'allegations'.

Kingdom, and the Investigating Committee of a National Board has taken the view that the offence leading to the conviction might be construed as misconduct of sufficient seriousness to necessitate removal of the right to practise. For the purposes of this legislation the term 'conviction' or the phrase 'convicted of a crime' applies only to those people who, having been found guilty, then have imposed upon them an actual prison sentence, a suspended prison sentence, a monetary fine or a Community Service Order. All other sentences (that is, a Probation Order, a conditional discharge or an absolute discharge) are prevented from being regarded as 'convictions' by section 13 of the Power of the Criminal Courts Act 1973. This does not mean that the Professional Conduct Committee cannot proceed in the matter – simply that they must hear some evidence as in the case of the true 'allegations', the procedure for which is illustrated in Figure 9.

Where the basis for the case to be heard is not a true 'conviction', the procedures must of necessity be more complex, since some facts must be established before the question of misconduct can be considered. While this is a relatively brief process where the respondent has been before a court and been found guilty of an offence (even though not 'convicted' for the purpose of subsequent proceedings), it can be extremely long and expensive where it involves hearing a large number of witnesses and concerns (for example) a number of alleged incidents in a hospital. You cannot, however, put a price on justice, so, no matter what the cost in time or money the witnesses must be heard. Such witnesses will be examined by the Council's solicitor, cross-examined by or for the respondent, and questioned by the Committee, all in order that the truth can emerge and the facts be established. (Figure 9 seeks to illustrate the procedures in diagrammatic form.)

The statutory rules are specific in respect of the nature and quality of evidence the Professional Conduct Committee must receive. This is no time or place for hearsay, imagination or fantasy. It is only concerned with fact which must stand up to challenge as if in a criminal court, and satisfy the same principles of natural justice. By the same token, it is not possible to refuse to attend to give evidence if called, since the UKCC has and uses powers of subpoena to compel attendance. The process is therefore strong and valuable from two standpoints. First, it is pointless to make allegations which question the appropriateness of a person to retain the right to practise if you cannot back those allegations with evidence which will stand a thorough questioning. Secondly, it provides a sound system for those who, in spite of pressure to the contrary from those in authority over them, express their professional concern and integrity by bringing allegations for which they have evidence.

As is the case with the Investigating Committees of the National Boards, the law (in the form of the Act and the statutory rules) prescribes the range of decisions available to the Professional Conduct Committee when it has established some facts, and considered that, in some culpable way, those facts are such as to be misconduct. Figure 10 indicates the available options.

Some aspects of Figure 10 require elaboration. It will be noted that one of the options available to the Committee is to postpone its judgement. Contrary to what some people say, to be made the subject of this decision is not to be 'let off'. The respondent will have to come back to a resumed hearing on a planned date with references and reports about the intervening period and face a Committee which still has the same options available to it – including that of removal from the register.

Another point to note is that the Committee, in deciding whether to

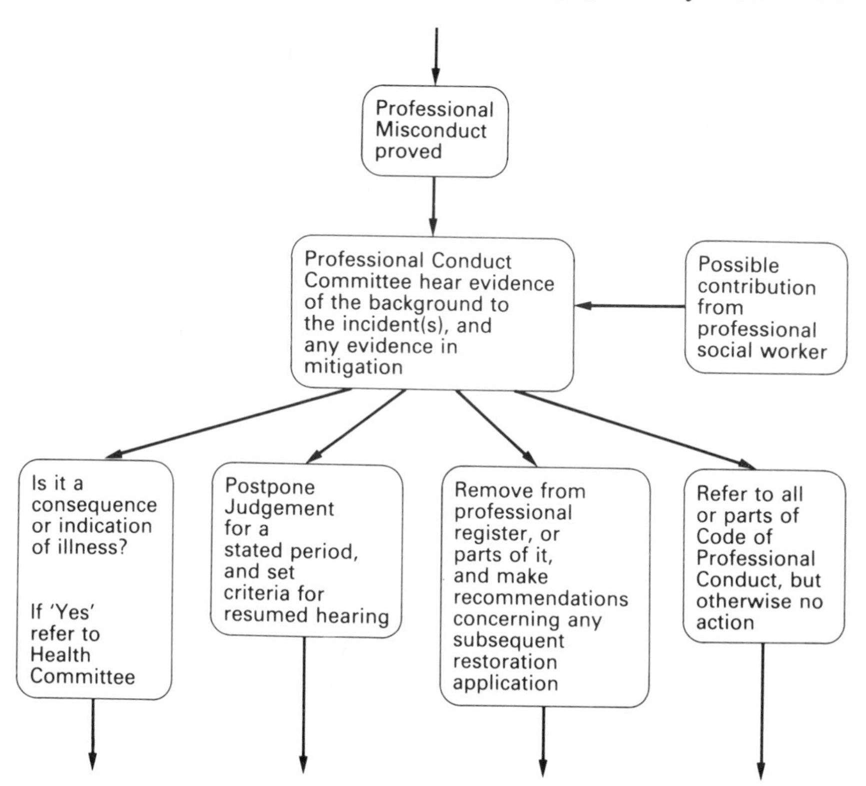

Figure 10. Decisions available to Professional Conduct Committee.

remove a person's name from the professional register, now has to decide whether that decision will apply to all parts or only some of the parts for which that person has professional qualifications.

Unlike the practitioner who is the subject of a postponement of judgement and who therefore must return to the Committee, the person who is removed from the register will only return if he or she makes an application for restoration. In contrast with the replaced legislation, the rules now state that an application for restoration will not be heard in the absence of the respondent unless there are overwhelming reasons for his or her absence. This is surely correct, in that it emphasises just how important is the decision to give back to someone the right to practise which was previously removed from them by reason of their proven misconduct. At the same time, the fact that the rules allow application for restoration, and that many successfully apply, indicates that removal is not necessarily the end of a person's professional career. Indeed, for many the day of removal is seen in retrospect as the day on which rehabilitation began.

This chapter must not come to an end without reference to the new procedures for considering alleged unfitness to practise where that unfitness is a consequence of illness, even though at the time of writing they are only just at the point of coming into operation.

The Nurses, Midwives and Health Visitors Act 1979 provided a legislative hook by allowing for 'removal for misconduct or otherwise'. The statutory rules made within that power allow that a person may be removed if 'her fitness to practise is seriously impaired by reason of her physical or mental condition'. The means by which such removal can be achieved is a procedure involving consideration by at least three nurse, midwife or health visitor members of the UKCC (the Professional Screeners), independent medical examinations, and a Health Committee made up of UKCC members.

It has been indicated in the parts of this chapter concerned with the Investigating and Professional Conduct Committees that their powers include that of referral to the UKCC Health Committee where, in their considered judgement, the matters with which they are faced are a consequence or indication of illness. While cases can be referred from those sources, they are not the only sources.

Just as it is any citizen's right (whether or not themselves a professional nurse, midwife or health visitor) to allege professional misconduct against a nurse, midwife or health visitor, so it is their right to raise a question as to whether a practitioner's fitness to practise is seriously impaired by reason of illness. The only difference is that, before any proceedings are initiated on the basis of such a question, the person raising it must make it in the form of a statutory declaration, since the end-result of the process being initiated may be removal of the right to practise.

As was indicated at the beginning of this chapter, this book has been written at a time of enormous change in the profession's statutory regulatory structures and associated procedures. For this very reason, it is impossible to illustrate it with examples of new case-law. It is, however, an incontrovertible fact that what we now have is legislation which goes further than that which it replaces in providing for the protection of the public.

More significant even than that is the fact that it also gives much more of the responsibility for the regulation of the profession to the profession's own members.

This legislation really is the framework within which the profession creates and operates the means of honouring its contract with society.

Chapter 10
Managing the Team

CHRISTINE HANCOCK

The concept of team management within the National Health Service was introduced formally as one of the key features of the 1974 Health Service reorganisation, that *multi-disciplinary management teams should be formed at each level to plan and coordinate the Health Service.* Interestingly, another key feature was identified as the active participation by clinicians in management. From 1974, formal management teams were set up at every level of the National Health Service and each team included an administrator, a nurse, a treasurer and a community physician. Regional teams also included the works officer, and district teams included a hospital consultant and a general practitioner chosen by their colleagues. The 1982 Health Service reorganisation continued the concept of team management. Teams exist to manage a complex service so that the views of all the major disciplines can be expressed and considered before a decision is taken. Part of the concern about the 1974 reorganisation was about the concept of team management, and particularly the concept of *consensus* management.

An organisation as complex as the National Health Service, and indeed many other large organisations, have to consider the views of many different departments – very few departments can function effectively in isolation. The operating theatre staff cannot decide alone to alter their pattern of working: they will affect the surgical wards, the cleaning schedules and maybe the staff canteen, pharmacy and pathology services, out-patient clinics and staff training programmes. The essentially integrating way in which teams work was reinforced by their collective responsibility to the health authority and by the requirement that their decisions must be by consensus. Each member of the team had the power of veto, making this particular definition of consensus the equivalent of unanimous agreement. Concern expressed about the management of the National Health Service in the late 1970s was not only about levels of management but also about the style of management and particularly about consensus management. Consensus management, it was alleged by many, led to slowness in decision-making and often to no decisions at all.

The Royal Commission on the National Health Service considered team decision-making and the members' report stated that decisions should be taken jointly on matters which are not exclusively the responsibility of any one member of the team and which are not covered in any approved plans nor regulated by established policies of the health authority. The report described the advantages of consensus as bringing a wider dimension to team decision-making, bringing in different points of view, allowing such different views to be debated and highlighting the impact of one set of factors upon others. It was also felt that this meant there was a stronger commitment to such decisions and therefore a more effective implementation of them. The disadvantages of consensus were also well documented: the clashes of personality which occurred, the domination of the team by one individual, the feeling that compromises had to be reached, and the tendency to ignore rather than grapple with difficult problems. Consensus management meant that district management teams always presented a united view when often it would be better for choices and options to be presented to the health authority. The report concluded that consensus may mean that decisions take longer to reach but, when reached, they may be better decisions and may be implemented more rapidly. The members of the Royal Commission, in their report, reminded their readers that consensus management is not totally new: it has always been necessary in the National Health Service, and in other large organisations, for those people who are responsible for particular services to be in general agreement with their colleagues in different disciplines about any decisions which directly affected their own responsibility. Before consensus management was dreamt of, no sensible group secretary would have tried to tell matron how to do her job! There was consultation and discussion then, as there has to be now. The members of the Royal Commission and others felt that there was a risk that consensus management may sap individual responsibility by allowing it to be shared: it is important that managers should not be prevented from managing the services for which they are responsible. Consensus management works best where individual team members have a firm grasp of the distinction between their individual responsibilities and the responsibilities of the whole team.

The deliberations of the Royal Commission clearly influenced government ministers and their staff, for the circular describing the new structure and management of the National Health Service says of the district management team:

In its joint responsibilities – formulation of advice to the authority on district-wide policies, priorities and programmes and determining how decisions of the authority should be implemented – the team will operate by consensus. *This does not mean seeking unanimity at all costs*; significant differences of view should be reported to the authority, officers will be accountable individually for the performance of their own functions as well as being responsible jointly as members of the management teams.

One of the major criticisms of the structure of the Health Service since 1974 (particularly from doctors) has been the difficulty of getting decisions made at the level of the hospital or community services. One of the key features of the 1982 reorganisation is that of maximum delegation of responsibility to units. The HMSO publication *Patients First* stated: '... there should be a maximum delegation of responsibility to hospital and community services level. For each major hospital, or group of hospitals, and associated community services, there should be an administrator and a nurse of appropriate seniority to discharge an individual responsibility in conjunction with the medical staff'. If health authorities want to see this concept of delegation carried out, they have to carefully plan their management arrangements below district level. Health authorities spent much of 1982 deciding how to fulfil the requirement that they divide their district into units of management. The way in which units have been established will determine the nature of any team arrangement. A unit of management has one administrator and one director of nursing services. Many so-called units do not have this arrangement, particularly large hospital services where there are instances of one administrator but two or three directors of nursing services. In all these cases, medical representation may be complicated and management arrangements will have to be clarified and understood.

No Department of Health circular has given any indication that there is any collective responsibility for matters arising within a unit nor how any such responsibility should be managed. The administrator, nurse and doctor for each unit do exist and will work together, and whether together they are called a team, a group, or anything else seems to some extent to be an argument over semantics. What is important is that there are clearly defined and understood relationships within the unit team, between the unit team and the district management team, and between the individual unit officers and the appropriate district officer. One of the first things a unit team has to do is to consider its membership. The core membership is one administrator, one nurse and one doctor; if there is more than one director of nursing services or director of nurse education within the unit, then additional nurses may be members of the team; should a representative of the district treasurer's department attend? And the unit works officer? Is one doctor adequate? And should a general practitioner be involved with a hospital unit team? Will a university representative attend as in teaching district management teams? There is definitely a need for a team of only three to five but with possibly the close involvement of two or three others. Some unit teams include a treasurer, others have more than one doctor so that there is clinical involvement of a significant specialty or institution. Some unit teams hold a regular meeting when they involve a larger number of people, paramedical professionals, social workers, junior doctors and even a nurse representative. The unit team has to decide on whether to have a chairman and who that should be, on the frequency of meetings and the organisation of the agenda and minutes. It is important that there is a formal structure to the work of the unit team but there is a great advantage, too, in unstructured time when ideas can be shared and conflicts resolved. It is most important that such informal meetings are not occasions when decisions get taken in secret.

The essential task of management in the National Health Service, and particularly of unit management, is to organise limited resources – human, physical and financial – so as to enable the community to be provided with the best possible standard and balance of care. The demands which are made on resources by medical staff in providing clinical care and treatment have to be reconciled one with another. Doctors are an important source of innovation, both in medical practice and in general approaches to care and treatment and their ideas must be evaluated and, where appropriate, translated into action by management. The medical membership of the unit team is crucial if the unit is to see that active participation by clinicians in management which was planned in 1974. If the medical contribution is to mean anything at all, it is up to the nurse and administrator to facilitate that medical participation and to know what they expect from the medical representatives. It is quite unrealistic for the unit team to expect the medical member to agree anything which will affect a colleague's service or to agree readily to the implementation of change in a colleague's service in opposition to his view. The unit team does, however, have the right to expect that their medical member will act as an ambassador for unit policies and will argue and explain such policies to his colleagues. The unit nurse and unit administrator would do well to consider generously any pattern of working which facilitates the most effective medical participation as this will, hopefully, lead to better decision-making and easier implementation of those decisions.

Nursing could learn from the strengths of the medical role in team management and the director of nursing services should consider the appropriate involvement of clinical nursing colleagues. Nurses bring a particular professional strength and perspective to team management: they tend to be practical people; they are often the people most able to consider the impact which decisions will have on patients and their families; they are most aware of the overall environmental needs of patients. However, the director of nursing services alone cannot always bring the best possible professional view to the unit team and must consider the overall manner in which nursing opinion and knowledge reaches the unit team. Nurses as a group are crucial to the successful operation of a hospital or community service: they see the overall activity of the service continuously at all hours, through all the days and in all seasons. They have a great deal of knowledge of how the system works, they know its strengths and weaknesses and they should have ideas for change and improvement. If this wealth of knowledge is harnessed, listened to and acted upon then services will improve. Too often, however, clinical nurses share the frustrations of their medical colleagues and are less able to have their voice heard where decisions are taken. Similarly, too, directors of nursing services are often involved in decisions which are difficult to implement because an overall nursing view has not reached the unit.

Directors of nursing services should develop a system and an approach whereby there is no discussion at the unit team on a clinical service without the director of nursing services talking to the most senior clinical nurse involved in that service and, on many occasions, that clinical nurse might attend the unit team for the appropriate discussion. Similarly, clinical nurses and other nurse managers must make sure that they convey their problems, difficulties and ideas to the director of nursing services in a constructive way. There are, and indeed there should be, ideas for change and innovation which are not always expensive. Also, a very good proposal exerts subtle pressure on the unit team to generate the necessary resources. The involvement of a wide range of nurses in some of the unit's deliberations will help in the overall standard of communications within the unit. Nurses can improve or worsen the participation of doctors in unit management. The working relationship and professional understanding between nurses and doctors is usually better at the working level of hospital ward or theatre, clinic or health centre than it is between doctors and nurse managers. Where relationships are difficult between nurse managers and medical staff, clinical nurses face an uncomfortable conflict of loyalty or find themselves hostile to one or the other. Where clinical nurses participate in nursing management decisions and in the deliberations and decisions of the unit teams, they can be instrumental in narrowing the gap between the unit team and the medical staff. The implementation of any decision of the unit team will almost always be made much easier if the nurses understand fully what is to be done and the reasoning behind the decision, even if it is an unpopular decision. This places a particular responsibility on the director of nursing services' position within the unit team.

The director of nursing services has a personal and individual responsibility for the management of the unit nursing service and for this he/she is accountable to the district nursing officer, although the other members of the unit team will also have a concern. Nursing is an essential part, and may be the most essential part, of the overall service to patients. If the unit team is concerned about the overall service to the patients and about the overall running of the unit, then all members of the team should be interested in the nursing service and nurses should welcome this. Working in a multidisciplinary team means explaining things more to others, and means exposing your weaknesses and sharing your problems and your triumphs, but it also means having the support of your colleagues in other disciplines. This has been recognised over the years by nurses and others working with this approach in geriatrics and psychiatry and it is interesting that hospital and sector management teams developed informally in these areas.

The largest single item of expenditure in the unit budget will be nursing and the unit team will certainly be interested in how this is being spent, especially at a time of financial retrenchment. Too many directors of nursing services are now paying the price for many years of professional isolation and defensiveness and now find that their unit team colleagues lack an understanding of nursing issues. It is difficult, but not impossible, to explain to other health service staff the intricacies of nurse training programmes and their effects on the service, the heavier workload generated by an elderly hospital population, the increased nursing requirement of a shorter length of patient stay, the nursing consequences of new medical techniques and the additional work of a small but mobile and difficult inner-city caseload. In return for sympathy and understanding (!) nurses must expect to be questioned on why so many nurses seem to be in wards and departments during times when the work is lightest, what theatre nurses do when lists finish early and why discharge into the community is difficult despite an increase in community nurses. Similarly, nurse managers should identify for their team colleagues the problems they face – theatre lists and clinics cancelled with little warning, wards staffed at weekends with few patients, day hospitals whose patients only attend for four hours.

Debate and discussion among nurses and their colleagues from other disciplines will not only lead to better understanding but will also stimulate ideas on the better organisation of services and the use of resources. More important still, however, is the need to explain and justify the use of resources. Nursing consumes between 20 and 30 per cent of the overall budget of most districts but for some units the proportion may be as high as 50 per cent. It is well known that the amount of nursing resources available to the same types of patients varies greatly, not only across the country but even within some districts. This makes many staffing levels difficult to justify in the absence of any objective measures of the effectiveness of different levels of nursing care and therapy. The National Health Service as a whole pays little attention to any form of quality assurance but nurses could lead the way. To date, nurses have dismissed much of the work undertaken by non-nurses into nursing workload and this has been because a work study approach has been seen as professionally unacceptable, but at the same time nurses have ignored the growing volume of nursing research. There are many measurements of performance available now to nurse managers: none of them is perfect but certainly they can be considered. In the absence of good measurements of nursing performance, crude ones will be used by treasurers and others – nursing cost per in-patient day, per case, per out-patient attendance, etc. Nurses need to widen the debate about nurse staffing and workload: to involve clinical nurses, to involve team colleagues and to involve other directors of nursing services. In particular, nurses must look more closely at measurements of the outcome of nursing intervention so that a case can be made for resources for nursing as opposed to physiotherapy, domestics or maintenance when this is appropriate.

The director of nursing services' role on the unit team is not confined to nursing but should be one of involvement in all matters which relate to the unit. In some matters, of course, the nurse will have more knowledge and interest than others. In particular, a nurse will have strong views about the support services. Problems of repairs and maintenance are a major source of friction in many hospital and community services. In the late 1960s, nurses gave away much of their responsibility for and involvement in so-called *non-nursing* duties. Now many ill patients are nursed in an environment which is noisy, too hot or too cold, and often far from clean. Food is too often inappropriate as it is ordered too far ahead, poorly served and inadequate for the patients' nutritional needs. Food and drink are cleared away from patients by staff who are not primarily concerned with observing what the patient has eaten. Nurses on unit teams now have an unrivalled opportunity to talk with their administrators and plan the delivery of support services which is appropriate to their unit. One of the first things a unit team should do is to discuss how they will find out the patients' view of the unit. In particular, they need to consider the initial reception which patients face when they first arrive at the unit: in the clinic, out-patient department, casualty or admissions area. Unit teams also need to consider the way telephones are answered and enquiries dealt with. Notices around clinics and hospitals also need reviewing to see whether they are accurate and whether they create the right impression of the unit. Admission booklets, appointment cards and other written information which is given or posted to patients are rarely seen by the unit team and yet are important to patients and in the impression which they give of the unit.

The unit team as a whole needs to review various policies which affect patients. Practices will exist about visiting times, about the visiting of and by children, about visiting on the day of operation and about waking times. It is unlikely that there needs to be a single unit policy but the unit team should know what is practised and should consider any practices which they think are not satisfactory. The team should consider regularly information about the service which is offered to patients such as the time they have to wait for admission for certain conditions, the time before an appointment can be obtained in each specialty, the time patients actually wait in clinics, casualty and out-patient departments. Some of this information is available routinely but some will have to be collected specially and it may be necessary to use a simple anecdotal approach of asking patients at irregular intervals. All members of the unit team have a responsibility, both collectively and individually, for the quality of care within their unit and, however busy, should consider these and other indicators of that quality at each unit team meeting. Finally, the unit team must always consider all indications of a shortfall in the standard of care to patients. The health authority should have a procedure for the investigation of complaints and untoward incidents. All members of the unit team should see each complaint and the results of any investigation. Similarly, the unit team should investigate any serious untoward incidents. In addition to the report of any particular complaints or incidents, the team should always consider any general lessons which can be learned from an enquiry into a particular matter.

Performance indicators are now under discussion in every district and most districts will be considering such indicators for each of their units. Where a district has two similar units, such indicators can form the basis for some useful comparisons; more often, comparison will have to be between units in more than one district. Many performance indicators under consideration are fairly crude and the nursing costs need careful and detailed checking: often, certain school of nursing, planning or occupational health posts are included in the costs of the hospital at which they are based; the costs of all nurses in training may also be allocated to a single hospital and not over the whole training area. Unit teams have a responsibility to monitor the performance and efficiency of their unit, and district management teams will want to see that this is done. There are many ways of doing this of which the DHSS performance indicators is one way but not necessarily the best. An analytical look at the work of the unit is vital but so too is a qualitative assessment and, to quote the author Peter Drucker, 'to go oneself and look is the only reliable feedback'.

Reorganisation of the National Health Service is harmful to many individuals and certainly is harmful to aspects of the whole service. In particular, communications are harmed by the turbulence of organisational change. Unit teams have to work hard at communication systems between the team members but this must not be at the expense of communications around the unit. Unit teams are a new concept and people will confuse the unit team with the district management team. There will be concern about items which are on the agenda and concern about items which are not on the agenda. The unit team can aid communications by involving all those most concerned before any item is discussed and by giving feedback on all decisions. The director of nursing services is a key person because nurses will be working in all parts of the unit and if they are well informed, most staff will be, too. The unit team has a particular responsibility to measure and monitor the effectiveness of its communications system and there are many methods and schemes for doing this.

Unit teams have a responsibility for the industrial relations within their unit. Each unit nurse and administrator has a part to play in the health authority's disciplinary, grievance and other personnel policies. There may be a unit joint staff committee as well as the district joint staff committee. District management teams and unit teams will have to consider very carefully how industrial relations matters are managed as trade unions will be quick to exploit confusion in this sphere. Everything that can be delegated to the unit should be, as difficulties are more likely to be resolved at that level. Staff organisations will often want to see as many matters as possible taken to the health authority and it will require a united approach from district and unit officers to prevent this. The director of nursing services will need to work closely with the district nursing officer so that they both know of difficult problems and do not worsen these by poor communications between themselves. National Health Service management of recent years has given a low priority to operational management compared with planning future services. It is important that this balance is redressed as it sometimes seems as though the whole National Health Service was reorganised so that coat hooks could be put on the back of doors and dripping taps stopped! However, planning *is* important and unit teams will want to be involved in the planning of the future of their unit and indeed the future of the district.

The pattern of units will determine to some extent the role each unit can play. Units of particular care groups, such as primary care, will probably have the responsibility to develop the district strategy for their particular service. Other units may not be able to plan in isolation from one or more units who manage similar services, but it will still be important for the unit to be involved in the planning. A real difficulty for the unit will be the involvement of all staff in the unit and particularly doctors and nurses. It is especially hard, but especially necessary, to plan services at a time of financial stringency. Directors of nursing services should consider how best to involve their nursing colleagues in the planning process. Too few district plans make reference to nursing, to nursing manpower or to nursing education. To develop a plan for mental health services should require a plan for recruiting and training community psychiatric nurses. In fact, most strategies for mental health require more nurses but planning documents rarely refer to increasing the number of registered mental nurses. Nursing education often crosses several units but plans will be needed for the changes proposed locally and nationally. Many districts are facing very different employment patterns and plans should include a strategy for the employment and deployment of all nursing staff. Capital and service developments too often fail because the nursing manpower is not planned at the same time.

Unit teams will, of course, spend much of their time on budgetary issues. Within the unit team it is likely that there will be general agreement within the group that the overall planning and setting of the unit budget should be a matter for the whole unit to debate and discuss, if not necessarily to agree. Certainly, any ideas and bids for development should be a matter for the whole unit team. Controversy over budgets is most likely to arise over the two issues of control and virement. The manager of the nursing budget is the district nursing officer who allocates part of the nursing budget to the director of nursing services who controls the expenditure of that budget. Changes within the district pattern of services are likely to occur only through changes in the distribution of nursing posts and it is unlikely that the district nursing officer would concede overall direction of nursing resources. However, the unit team will also wish to consider the overall unit resources and how best to deploy them. Principles have to be agreed by the district, and the district management team and unit team must work at agreeing the detail.

Team management is not a simple concept, but management of the National Health Service is not simple! Unit management is very new and the challenges, opportunities, problems and difficulties have yet to be seen over time. Unit teams give directors of nursing services a marvellous opportunity to work with medical and administrative colleagues to plan and manage the overall service to patients. If nurses are really interested in improving the care of patients, this is their opportunity. To grasp such an opportunity, directors of nursing services must work from a position of knowledge and strength, they must represent nurses throughout the unit and ensure that nurses know how their views are represented. Additionally, directors of nursing services should work as a nursing team with the district nursing officer so that a nursing team develops which shares an overall nursing perspective of the district.

POSTSCRIPT

Since this chapter was prepared, the report of the NHS Management Inquiry has been published. The inquiry team, under the chairmanship of Mr Roy Griffiths, recommended radical change for the management of the NHS.

The report suggests the appointment of general managers, who may be nurses, at every level of the service. The report argues that without a general manager there is no driving force in the service.

At central government level the report recommends the establishment of a Health Service Supervisory Board, involving the Secretary of State and the Health Minister. Working to this supervisory board will be an NHS Management Board, involving high-level experts from within the service and a large number of non-NHS people, drawn from industry and commerce. The report also suggests the appointment of a national Director of Personnel Management.

There can be little doubt that the report of the NHS Management Inquiry will have widespread effects on the management arrangements pertaining to the NHS, but it will not alter the fact that in an organisation as large, complex and diverse as the NHS, consensus will be required for effective functional management on a day-to-day basis.

In this respect, this chapter remains valid. It is too early to predict the organisational change that the Griffiths Report will bring about, but whatever the structure, nurses will still be the largest professional group within the service. It follows that the nursing service will continue to need high-quality management by appropriately trained nurses. Those nurses engaged in management will continue to work in a team setting and need to understand what is involved in relating to other managerial disciplines.

Suggested further reading

DHSS (1980) *Circular HC(80)8. Health Service Development – Structure and Management.*

DHSS (1983) *Report of the NHS Management Inquiry* (Griffiths Report).

Ham, C. (1984) *Saving lives or saving money? The two crises of the NHS.* A paper prepared for a conference on the NHS, 'Crisis in Perspective', held at Guy's Hospital, 6 January 1984.

King's Fund (1977) *Decision Making in the New National Health Service – Consensus or Constipation?*

King's Fund (1982) *Unit Management in Context.*

Klein, R. (1983) *The Politics of the NHS.* London: Longman.

Management Arrangements for the Reorganised NHS (1972). London: HMSO.

Patients First (1979) London: HMSO.

Royal Commission on the National Health Service (July 1979) London: HMSO

Index